THE JOY OF SEXUAL FANTASY

This book is a companion volume to Dr Stanway's THE ART OF SENSUAL LOVING and is similarly addressed to couples who want to find out more about their own sexuality, in order to enhance their relationships. It is derived from the author's long clinical experience as a psychosexual and marital therapist, and is based on the sexual fantasies of his patients.

Everyone fantasizes, but not always consciously. Dr Stanway begins by examining the nature of fantasy – what fantasies are, their origins, and why people fantasize. He explains the universal human need to escape, at times, from reality, and shows how sexual and erotic fantasies have a therapeutic value.

Submission, showing off, romance, prostitution, nongenital love-making, fetishism, pain and *masochism* are among the 40 or more themes presented in Part Two, a comprehensive encyclopedia of fantasies. Each entry recounts a typical thematic fantasy from the author's case histories, and includes an analysis of what the fantasy tells its creator about his or her sex life. You can use Part Two as a reference section, in which to look up your favourite fantasy; and you can learn from the accompanying discussion of the theme what the fantasy has to tell you about your sexuality and that of your partner, and how this knowledge can be of value to you.

Practical tips and advice on how to enrich your fantasy life and how to use it to benefit your relationship are the subjects covered in the final part of the book. Readers who claim not to be able to fantasize are taken, step by step, through the author's own technique for increasing his patients' ability to fantasize; and couples with rich fantasy lives learn how to attain deeper levels of communication by sharing their fantasies.

Dr Stanway's frank and informative text is complemented perfectly by sensitive and beautiful color illustrations.

THE JOY OF SEXUAL FANTASY is essential reading for those keen to gain greater insight into their own and their partner's sexuality, and to use their understanding to benefit themselves and their relationships.

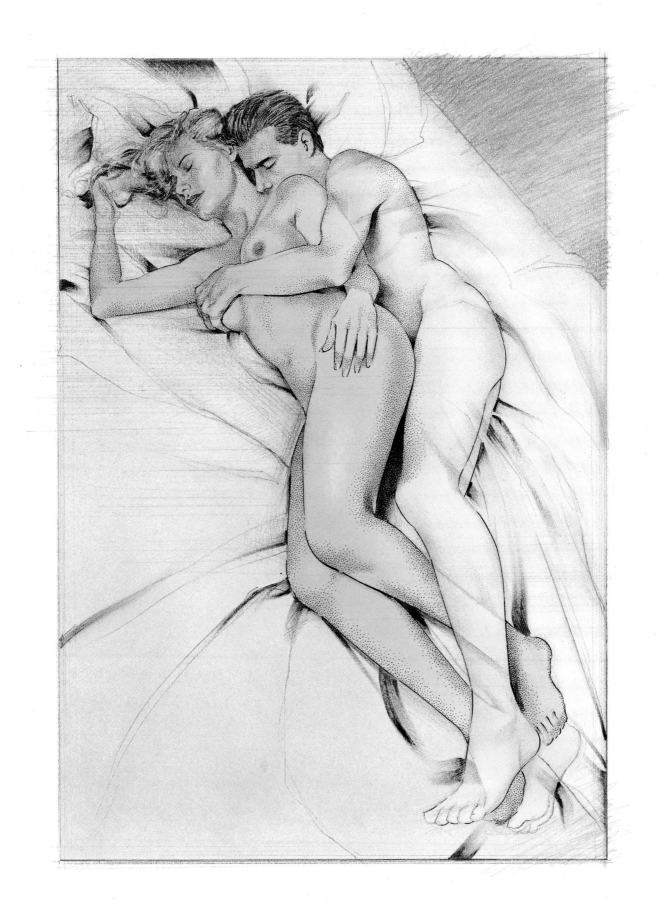

THE JOY OF SEXUAL FANTASY

DR ANDREW STANWAY

ILLUSTRATED BY JOHN GEARY

Carroll & Graf Publishers, Inc.
New York

Text copyright © Andrew Stanway 1991
Illustrations copyright © Eddison Sadd Editions 1991
This edition copyright © Eddison Sadd Editions 1991

The right of Andrew Stanway to be identified
as author of this work has been asserted by him
in accordance with the British Copyright.
Designs and Patents Act 1988.

All rights reserved

First published in the United States in 1991
by Carroll & Graf Publishers, Inc.

Carroll & Graf Publishers, Inc.
260 Fifth Avenue
New York, NY 10001

Fourth printing 1995

Library of Congress Cataloging-in-Publication Data
Stanway, Andrew
    The joy of sexual fantasy / by Andrew Stanway:
illustrated by John Geary
        p.   cm.
    ISBN 0−88184−S52−X : $15.95
    1. Sex customs.   2. Sexual fantasies.   I Title
HQ21.5625   1991
306.77--dc20   90−20780
                                                    CIP

AN EDDISON · SADD EDITION
Edited, designed and produced by
Eddison Sadd Editions Limited
St Chad's Court
146B King's Cross Road
London WC1X 9DH

Phototypeset by Bookworm Typesetting,
Manchester, England
Origination by Columbia Offset, Singapore
Produced by Paramount Printing Company, Hong Kong

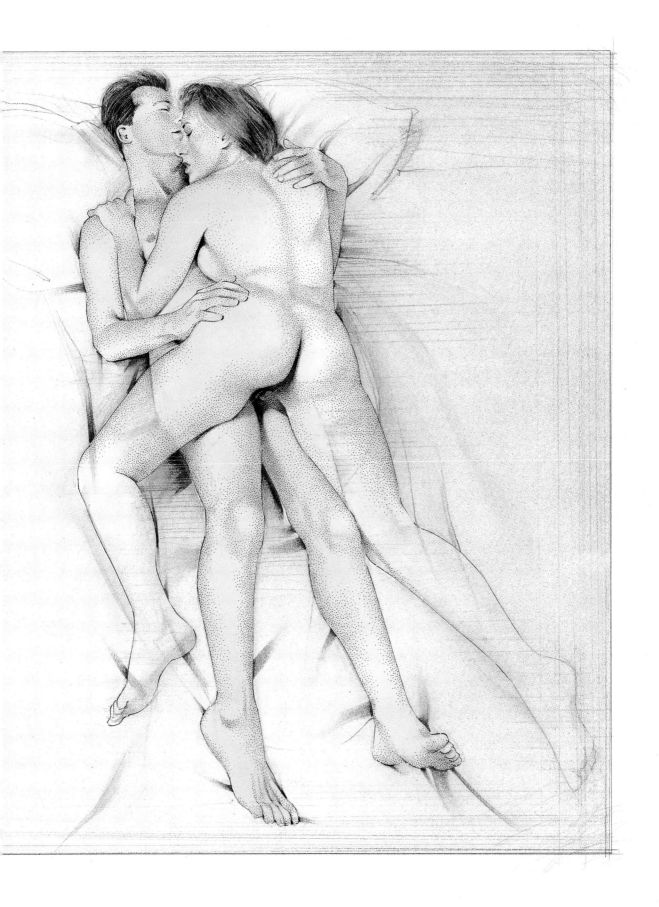

DEDICATION
To everyone who has been brave enough to
share their innermost secrets with me.
I hope that by being a good custodian I
can in some way help others to help
themselves . . . and by doing so,
enable those who have put their trust
in me to bring reassurance, understanding
and sexual delight into the lives
of my readers.

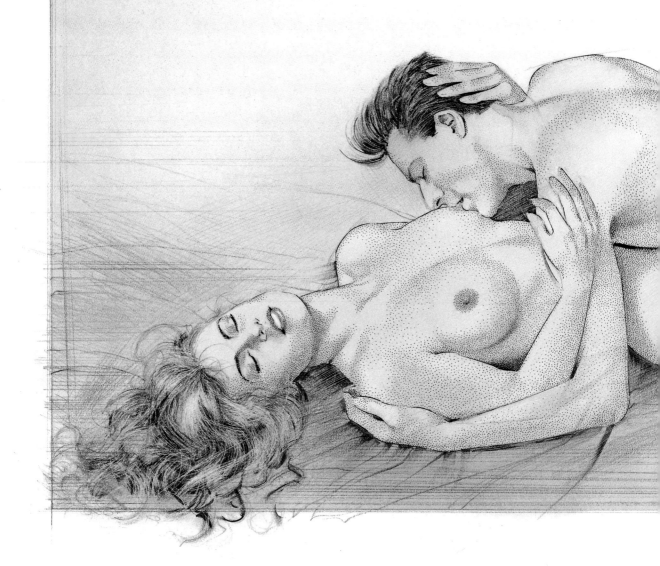

CONTENTS

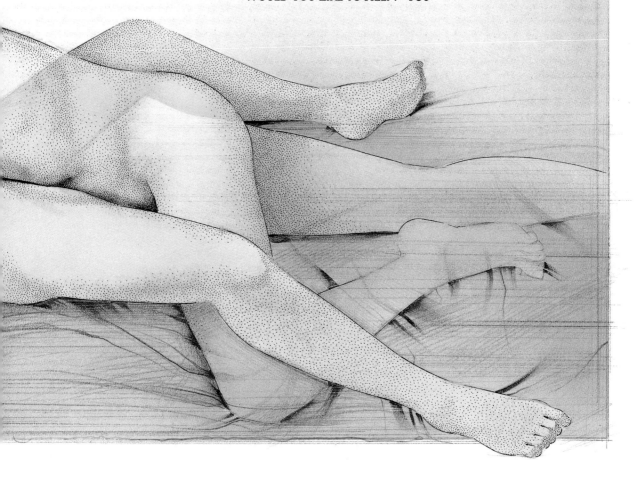

FOREWORD

The proper study of Mankind is Man
(Alexander Pope 1688–1744)

Since I qualified in medicine in the sixties, the subject of erotic fantasies has become acknowledged as something worthy of consideration by professionals and non-professionals alike. Until the mid-sixties, apart from the work of Kinsey published nearly twenty years before, in which fantasies were mentioned among a whole mass of human sexual behaviour, little appeared in the professional press on this practically universal human experience.

That which did start to appear in the sixties largely dealt with fantasy as a manifestation of the 'ill' mind . . . drawing, no doubt, on similar views expressed by Freud and some of his followers.

In 1973 a leading US 'expert' wrote in *Cosmopolitan* that 'women do not have sexual fantasies'. Just two years later another psychiatrist refuted this crazy notion with the contention that 'all women have sexual fantasies'. Confusion abounded in the professional mind.

When researching the learned literature to write this book I unearthed nearly 300 papers on the subject of erotic fantasy. Clearly the subject has come of age since the early seventies and now few people are surprised to learn that most of us fantasize and that increasing numbers of us accept our fantasy life and make it a rich part of our sexual and non-sexual lives.

I spend on average about fifteen hundred hours a year listening to people's sexual and marital problems – and have done so for some years. Getting people to talk about their erotic fantasies is not easy, and any study of the subject is dogged by the internal censor that automatically comes into play as one human being recounts his or her innermost thoughts to another. I realize, therefore, that what I am told may not be the whole 'truth' . . . whatever that means, but outside the therapy room there are very few places where most of us feel at all free to share our fantasies. Not only is the relationship between therapist and client a specially privileged one that is based on openness and trust, but in a practice such as mine, much of what my patients impart to me arrives in my unconscious or conscious in ways that go beyond simply talking and listening.

Among the most profound lessons I have learned with my patients – and the things that have led to the greatest improvements in their insights, understanding and behaviour – involve non-verbal techniques using body-mind manoeuvres and regression to childhood and even beyond. There are no actors and actresses in these sessions – nobody kidding anybody about anything – simply two human beings walking the stony path to a realization of what lies in the patient's mind and soul.

This sort of therapy is hard work for both client and therapist, but the results it yields are formidable. Dreams flow, drawings and paintings emerge, poetry comes 'from nowhere' and so on as the conscious mind starts to come to terms with the wonders revealed from the depths of the unconscious.

Obviously, readers of this book are not 'patients', and I have no intention of treating them as such. However, we are all human and there is ample evidence to show that the people I see are much the same as everyone else when it comes to sexual fantasies. Several studies have shown that only about three per cent of all those with sexual difficulties consult a professional about them. This leaves millions who do not. And this doesn't take into account those of us who have no such problems, yet have fantasies as a normal part of our everyday life. I say this because although I see people with 'problems', the learned medical and psychological literature now abounds with studies of thousands of ordinary people off the street whose experience is just like those I see. Sexual fantasies are not, and never have been the preserve of the sexually 'ill' or 'odd'. They are universal, whether they are consciously acknowledged or not.

That our fantasies are so universal is partly due to the formidable power of modern-day media – a greatly underestimated force in the creation and maintenance of sexual and erotic fantasies. It was simply a matter of time before entrepreneurs discovered ways of making even more money from our fantasies – telephone sex lines now supplement hard and soft porn to add further millions to the industry's coffers. At a time when safe sex is high on the agenda the erotic fantasy industry in all its forms offers just about the safest sex there is: sex in the mind. It is bound to flourish.

THE JOY OF SEXUAL FANTASY falls into three sections. In Part One: **What Are Fantasies?** I look at the most common questions that I have been asked over the years as a therapist and as an Agony Uncle in women's magazines. Part Two: **Understanding Your Fantasies**, describes and analyzes more than 40 of the most common fantasies that occur in the Western world. Of course you won't find every specific fantasy mentioned and this is hardly surprising, given the enormous creativity of the human mind, but few themes are left out. In this part of the book I try to explain the psychological and emotional background to each fantasy type in ways that could help any couple understand one another better.

Part Three: **Learning to Fantasize**, goes through some practical areas that I have found helpful. I feel it is wrong to enlarge someone's vision, and then to give him or her a telescope that looks at things only one way. This last section should enable you to turn the telescope around and see things differently for you and your partner.

I say 'for you and your partner', not because I see sexual fantasies as something that we have only with or in the context of, our partner – though we might – but because fantasies are such a rich ground in which to grow the seeds of insight and knowledge. In this way most of us can, with some effort, improve our one-to-one relationships beyond recognition. Our fantasies often supply us with answers that we could come by in no other way short of formal 'therapy' of some kind. And in an age of AIDS, with newly fashionable concepts of long-term fidelity, anything we can do to enrich our sexual lives will lead to greater fulfilment over many years of monogamy.

Sexual fantasies, then, are powerful tools if properly and responsibly used. I hope that by the end of the book you'll have not only more tools in your box, but that you will also be skilled at using them for your own benefit and that of your relationship.

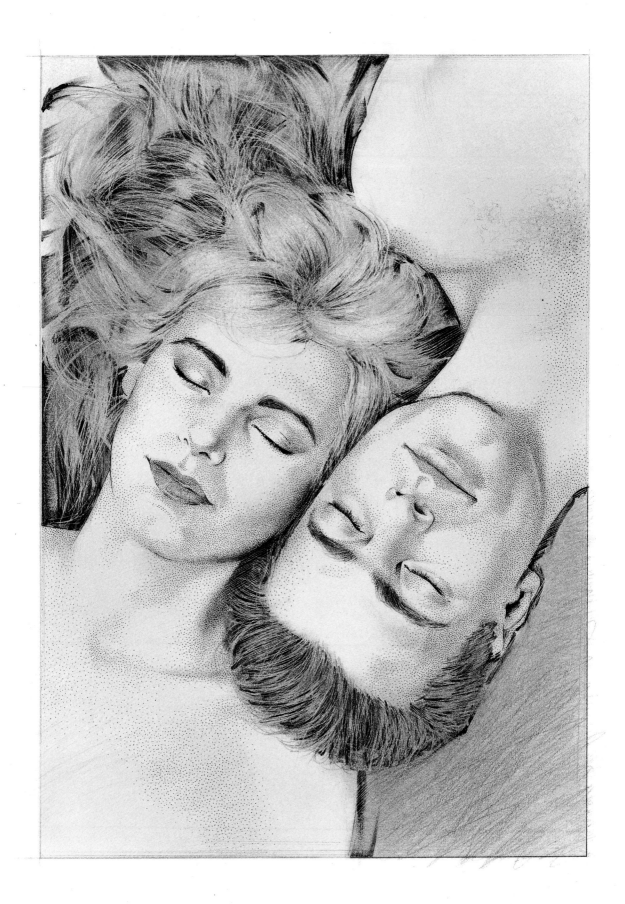

PART ONE

WHAT ARE FANTASIES?

Sexual fantasy is a complex area of human experience. While some people aren't even sure what a fantasy is, the link between dreams, fantasies and day-dreams, and whether such experiences are normal, are questions that fascinate some people and baffle others. Some questions recur time and again as people try to understand what fantasies are and how their fantasies relate to those of their partners and others. This chapter deals with these questions.

Sexual and erotic fantasies are almost certainly a universal part of human experience. Some people claim not to have any fantasies, but this doesn't mean that they can't have them.

The earliest specific references to sexual fantasies date back to the twelfth century, but the ancients certainly knew of their existence. Little is known about fantasies in ancient times, because the matter was not studied in the way it is today. However, there can be little doubt that many of the myths that survive to this day – Oedipus is the obvious example – and probably others that don't, had their origins in those areas of the mind that create frank sexual fantasies. The way in which various generations through the ages articulated the deepest recesses of their unconscious varied according to what was socially acceptable, but the key psychic processes that were taking place were much the same as those in today's fantasies. There's little, if any, evidence that people have changed much in their basic needs and desires over many centuries.

In the twelfth century fantasies were said to be visitations from supernatural beings; the male was called an 'incubus' and the female a 'succuba'. These other-worldly beings were thought to inhabit or visit the sleeping or day-dreaming individual's body temporarily, to bring sexual experience not based on reality. In the sixteenth century writers referred to such visitations as a manifestation of disease. Even as late as 1904, Havelock Ellis, the distinguished author of *Studies in the Psychology of Sex*, described the case of a girl who thought her fantasies were caused by demon possession.

If little has been written in history about sexual fantasies, and only during the last 25 years has the subject been studied seriously and systematically, it's understandable that little has been done to compare the ways in which various peoples around the world use fantasy. It seems self-evident that different cultures would produce different fantasies, but I've been able to find only one study that documents this really well. Research carried out in 1983 by the Institute of Psychiatry, London and the University of Hyogo, Japan, found that British men had twice as many fantasies as Japanese men; and Japanese women a quarter those of British women.

The survey questioned 60 men and 71 women, all Japanese student teachers at university. They were given a Japanese translation of a questionnaire, previously used to great effect in the UK. The study compared and contrasted the answers to the same questions being asked to these two populations. On four aspects of sexual fantasy: 'participating in an orgy'; 'giving oral sex'; 'being whipped or spanked'; and 'being aroused by watching someone urinate', no Japanese women reported experiencing any fantasies.

Perhaps the Japanese are more reserved than the British. Although foreigners hear much of Japanese brothels, prostitution services and outrageous television shows, the fact is that as a society, Japan is highly moral, somewhat puritanical and sets much store by family life. Perhaps the fantasy life of the Japanese will take some years to catch up with the very considerable changes occurring in their conscious attitudes to sexuality. However, given the considerable creativity of the Japanese and the many Western models of sex they could adopt, the nature of Oriental fantasy will undoubtedly change.

FANTASIES, DREAMS AND DAY-DREAMS

The biggest single step forward in the understanding of fantasies came with Freud and his exploration of the unconscious. Others before him had talked of a part of the mind that was not under conscious control. He and his followers refined these concepts and created the base on which our current understanding of fantasy is built.

Freud uses the word 'fantasy' in many different ways, to include both conscious day-dreams and their unconscious counterparts. Conscious day-dreams are things people dream up while awake. They are clearly under some sort of conscious control because the dreamer can start and stop them as required. But the content is only partly under conscious control; the unconscious plays its part, too. If you come to believe a day-dream is reality, it's called a hallucination or a delusion.

Day-dreams probably help make up – in the realm of conscious thought – for insufficient gratification in real life. In this way they can be used as a defence against unacceptable realities in everyday life.

No one knows what happens in the brain to produce fantasies. Certain psychological diseases are accompanied by hallucinations or delusions, the best-known being schizophrenia. Drugs, or a very high fever, can cause hallucinations. One group of drugs, the benzodiazepines, of which the best-known example is Valium, produces erotic sexual hallucinations in a tiny proportion of those who are given it intravenously. This was first discovered by dentists, who used the drug to sedate anxious patients before major dentistry. In several well controlled situations, allegations of sexual arousal and subsequent abuse were made by women against dentists, yet witnesses maintained that nothing in fact took place.

When I use regression techniques in my practice, my patients go into a sort of hypnotic trance, or state of altered consciousness, in which they see very clearly certain situations which took place in the past and which, under normal conditions, they would be unable to recall. They're perfectly conscious. In fact one woman, vividly reliving a particularly painful, previously forgotten, part of her childhood, complained because the barking of my dog outside the window disturbed her recollections.

How people see situations in the mind's eye with such clarity in health and disease is not understood, but see them they certainly can and do. Individual ability to do this varies a great deal, but almost everyone can be trained to improve the skill of calling to mind real, fictional or remembered events from the past.

DREAMS OF DELIGHT

Day-dreams share many properties with nocturnal dreams. Both to some extent aim to fulfil the dreamer's innermost wishes; and both allow a link to be made between innermost psychological needs and what the world around can actually provide. A day-dream thus involves a current impression which arouses a wish. It recalls past experiences of satisfaction and creates a promise of future delights as the original wish is fulfilled.

Freud suggested that some fantasies and day-dreams come from the unconscious and others from a slightly more available part of the mind, the pre-conscious. He claimed that fantasies are ways of relating to old psychic material in a way the conscious mind can tolerate. But as soon as things get tough, the fantasy is pushed into the unconscious and the original wish that triggered it has to find an alternative outlet, perhaps as a neurotic symptom.

So, according to Freud, conscious fantasy or day-dreaming is a reaction to a frustrating external reality. The imagination creates a wish-fulfilling situation in the mind to reduce the tensions created by the frustrating reality. The fantasist is aware that the reverie is unreal, but it serves its purpose and can be called upon again, when reality again starts to cause pain.

Not all fantasies are available to the conscious mind. In response to frustrating situations, people can also create unconscious fantasies that are no less powerful. This is especially true in dream life in which there's a high degree of organization and symbolism to protect people from the reality of their difficult, unconscious processes. Freud went on to elaborate this material with increasing complexity over many years, but for most people today there are other ways of looking at fantasy. To me, the term 'sexual fantasy' encompasses the complex conscious and unconscious day-dreams people have or the unwitting meaning they attach to certain ways of behaving. Sexual fantasies are not the same as erotic nocturnal dreams, which are outside conscious control, nor are they totally within a person's conscious control. All of this makes the definition of fantasy very difficult, yet most people think they know what they mean when they talk of their own fantasies.

WHY DO PEOPLE FANTASIZE?

Right from their earliest days as babies, people try to make sense of reality as they perceive it. When they can't explain something, they make up theories that appear to fit the world as they see it. For example, a very young girl may see a pregnant woman and, thinking that she became fat by eating, as most people do, theorize that pregnancy comes about as a result of eating too much. This theory now colours her play and fantasies and seems completely reasonable to her, given her knowledge of the world. Similarly, a three-year-old boy may well reason that babies come out of a mother's behind (anus) simply because this is the only place he is aware of that allows internal objects (faeces) to gain access to the outside world. Such theories then become a sort of reality that forms the basis for the child's fantasies. They are usually perfectly conscious explanations that the child will, if asked, elaborate with conviction.

Other personal theories are not so easily elicited from a child. These have been squashed by the conscious mind because they cause too much pain. For example, I see many individuals who believe that their genitals are dirty or sinful. They cannot say why they feel like this, they have no conscious belief that their genitals are unacceptable, yet they feel terrible when asked to touch them and become anxious even when they talk about doing so. Such adults are often plagued by unconsciously held theories about genitalia, usually taken directly from their parents. In this sense, sexual and erotic fantasies are no different from any others; they are transferred direct from the unconscious of the adult to that of the child.

Unlike the consciously held theories of childhood, such beliefs are not easily amenable to change in the face of new knowledge. A child who has learned about the existence of the vagina no longer needs to theorize that babies come out of the back passage, and the old theory is discarded. Unconsciously held beliefs are, however, dismissed less easily; many people take them to the grave. Such unconscious early theories can dominate an adult's sexual life. An individual may, unconsciously, equate the anus with sexual expression, while knowing that the vagina is the female genital organ of receptive pleasure.

Fantasies may date back even further than earliest conscious or unconscious theories about sex. Many philosophers and psychologists have suggested that everyone shares a sort of collective unconscious which affects sexual fantasy life, among other things. An example of this can be seen in fantasies that some children have of their parents making love. Even very young children, who have never seen or heard their parents having sex, can have such fantasies, often in considerable detail. Children raised in nurseries with no opportunity of observing adult sexual encounters play sexually with one another in ways that could not have been learned. A similar notion is that of the 'devouring' or 'biting' vagina: in many cultures throughout the world myths exist of vaginas that bite off a man's penis. Given that such cultures have never commented on the matter, the stories are either completely haphazard coincidence, which seems unlikely, or form part of a collective memory among humans. That these myths are so universal in human communities adds further evidence to support the idea of the inheritance of beliefs, theories and ways of behaving.

It certainly makes sense to me that babies might start fantasizing in the womb, as soon as they can link their emotions and their thinking to a sense of self. Just when this occurs is open to doubt, but work that I, and therapists like me, do in taking people back to intra-uterine experiences shows that they can remember far more than most of the medical and psychological fraternity would ever think possible. Such remembered stories can be verified by talking to the individual's mother. All of this makes me certain that a baby in the womb is already learning about the outside world and is undoubtedly forming links between feelings and what appears to produce them. It's not known for how many months this process occurs before birth, but it's naïve to suggest that a baby starts to try to make sense of his or her environment only at birth.

I should point out that although this book is about sexual fantasies, most people have fantasies about many other subjects, most of which come about as a result of much the same psychic processes as I describe here. What makes sexual fantasies so fascinating and revelatory is that they often relate back to various primitive developmental stages in life, when a person was faced with the assorted psychosexual tasks that have to be undertaken and absorbed in order to become a successful sexual adult. Sexual intercourse, and all human love-making, is a somewhat regressive process. In every erotic encounter, real or in the mind, people journey back into adolescence, childhood and babyhood in varying degrees and in different ways. The courtship of adolescence, the masturbation and self-centred stages immediately following puberty, the parent-love of pre-school years and the oral, anal and genital erotic stages that precede this Oedipal stage from birth, are all enacted in many different, often barely disguised ways that become a familiar part of adult love play. Sexual fantasies are simply the revealed psychic part of this story and serve a similar function. In a sense they are a kind of adult psychic play.

A patient of mine serves to illustrate this point rather well. He found that he was drawn in his fantasies to rubber, particularly the rubber pants that go over babies' nappies (diapers). In his conscious mind he couldn't explain why this should be and he was asked to see me because the police became involved with his behaviour as he tried to touch children's pants while they were wearing them. He was not in any sense a child molester. He was interested only in the rubber pants, not the child inside them. He had even bought a pair of rubber pants to use as a fetish object when masturbating.

In therapy it became clear that when this patient was very young his highly obsessional mother used to lie him on a rubber sheet in bed, just in case he wet the sheets. Hundreds of hours in the company of this rubber sheet made him come to see it as a sort of mother substitute, much as children have their 'cuddlies' - bits of blanket or cloth that they use as what psychologists call transitional objects. A child, in the absence of real love and care from a parent, forms a meaningful attachment to such an object (in my patient's case the rubber sheet), and craves it whenever life becomes difficult. For much of his life my patient was a well adjusted, successful family man, but when his unconscious was triggered he regressed to needing his love object – the rubber smell and texture. This gave him true satisfaction and a sense of being loved.

None of this was apparent to him when he first came to see me, and the meaning of his fantasies about rubber pants was obscure, to put it mildly. No doubt as he discovered his penis and its erotic potential in childhood he came to masturbate as a little boy, perhaps at first to comfort himself on the many long occasions he spent alone and lonely in bed, feeling abandoned by his controlling and rigidly unloving mother. By doing so he came to associate sexual arousal with the smell and feel of the rubber sheet, and then became unable to function without it. The result of this was a marital relationship that left a lot to be desired sexually, and eventual divorce.

PLAY-ACTING

Childhood games are a most fertile ground for learning how to fantasize. Infants spend a great deal of their time playing, and fantasy play is a common activity among children of every society. Fantasies – at the heart of most children's games – sow the seeds for creativity in later life. Much music, art and theatre is only a form of structured child's-play fantasy created for a society that rewards those who can use fantasy skills practised in childhood to please others. Good story-tellers, for example, have been cherished, even revered, in almost every culture throughout history.

Much can be learned about adult sexual fantasy from watching children at play. How many times do children say, 'I was only playing. It was just a game. It doesn't mean anything,' when trying to disavow the implications of a game? Children reassure themselves that playtime, like the play on a stage, comes to an end, or can be broken off at will. Games are controllable, unlike real life. An activity ceases to be play, however, when it can't be stopped at will. This has important implications for adult compulsive fantasies. Some adult perversions appear to come about when a highly specialized childhood plot becomes so ingrained in the unconscious that it remains necessary to the working of the psyche. Many people with perversions say they need a very detailed and consistent plot line if they are to enjoy their fantasy. One small change to the plot can reduce the fantasy's appeal or its ability to arouse.

In the context of fantasy development, the term 'playing with yourself' can be seen to have all kinds of symbolic meaning. From very early in life people start to play with notions of their sexuality. They pick up from their parents and other key adults a whole mass of data about sex, much of it contradictory. To try to make sense of it, they create game situations that may or may not be played with other people. Much of the doctor-nurse, 'I'll show you mine if you show me yours' games of young childhood are an effort to make at least some sense of this mass of information. Even trying to find out is highly charged emotionally because it conflicts with some of what has already been learned.

Classic psychoanalytical thought has it that the majority of fantasies arise from trying to cope with the traumas experienced right from the very first days of life. Life doesn't go without a hitch for most people. From the start, painful situations must be faced: a young baby has to endure being left in need of a feed while the telephone is answered; a child may feel neglected by an ill or busy mother, or unfairly punished by an angry parent. Any form of parental behaviour that inspires strong feelings creates, or has the ability to create, a corresponding fantasy.

CONFUSING REALITY

A further problem is that little babies and young children have the greatest difficulty making distinctions between reality as perceived by themselves and as perceived by others. Because of this they may see a mother as evil and hateful if she doesn't come to feed them when they are hungry, and fear they will die if she doesn't answer their needs. When she does come, they see her as good, and dare not show any hate for her for fear she might actually leave.

But this mountain of ill feeling against her cannot be so easily dispelled and, as a result, children often turn it inward, deducing that it must have been something to do with the way they are that she didn't come and look after them in the first place. Now, instead of seeing the mother as bad – an unacceptably dangerous idea – the child becomes 'bad' to absolve her. It is not hard to see that many traumas such as these can, with time and repetition, create an internal reality in a baby which has little or nothing to do with reality as perceived by the adult world. Nevertheless, this reality is true for the baby, who starts to create fantasies around it.

It will be useful here to take a brief look at the concept of reality. Material reality is obviously that which is provable to anyone by the use of their senses. But scientifically speaking, reality is anything that truly exists and is objective, whether perceived or logically inferred. This distinguishes the discovered from the invented, fact from theory, and existential reality from contrived fantasy. By this definition the functions of the mind, and the drives to be fed, to have sex, and so on, are not imagined, but real experiences.

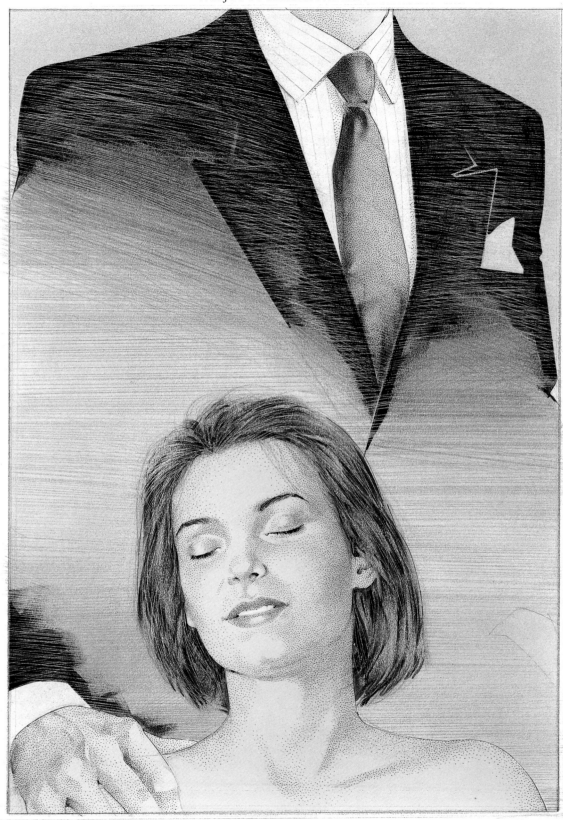

Because an individual is regularly discovering and rediscovering reality, it will always be unknowable; and perceptions of reality are subject to change as time passes. For babies, the concept of reality is bounded by the sensory functions they bring to bear on the subject in hand. Few babies and young children are brought up to use all their sensory faculties in equal measure; I suspect, for example, that the vast majority have less emotional and psychic stimulation than they could easily deal with.

What adults offer their children greatly affects how the young perceive the world, how they interpret it, and how they fantasize about it. Many parents deny their children's reality, by denying the truth of their statements; for example the child says, 'I'm afraid,' and Mother says, 'No you're not.' In doing so, all of this development becomes even more tricky.

In addition to all this perceived reality in children are the imposed truths of the particular society in which they live. From the moment of birth – even before – philosophical, political, religious, ethical, scientific, moral and other notions are woven into the story, all of which complement or conflict with what children see as their own world.

A considerable clinical problem, which can be highly confusing for some individuals, arises when trying to distinguish between fact and fantasy. For example, I sometimes see a woman who doesn't know whether or not she was sexually molested in her childhood. Her fantasy is all too real, but she can't resolve in her mind whether the fantasy arose from some kind of real experience or whether she made it all up. Given the power of the unconscious to embroider sexual matters it can, indeed, be almost impossible to decide, outside long-term therapy, where the truth lies. Questions of fact or fallacy can, however, be purely academic in many such cases, because the fantasy is often so real it might just as well have been fact. Distinguishing the two may never be possible, but the individual still has somehow to deal with the results of the experience, real or imaginary, if it is troubling her.

WORKING IT OUT

As children grow in the pre-school years these factors come together as they try to make some sort of sense of them. When the going gets tough many children, and indeed adults, regress to previous stages of their emotional development in order to try to recap, as it were. Much of this regression occurs at the unconscious level and is unplanned. However, in play and fantasy, people try to deal with the difficulties that assault them even though the original system that caused the hurt is long gone and can't be dealt with in reality. All fantasy is simply a way of acting out in the mind a scenario that makes life acceptable now, when life in the past was unacceptable in some way.

Story, myth and legend all have similar origins to sexual fantasy. Every character in depictions as apparently different as fairy tales, pantomimes, Greek myths, and James Bond films have more in common than many people

Issues of power, authority and control are never far away in sexual encounters. This woman's fantasy of her powerful boss, with all his wealth, excites her in a way that nothing else can.

realize. It has been said that Greek mythology told every story there was to be told. In a profound sense this is true. Human beings have battled with psychic monsters, unloving mothers and absent fathers since time immemorial, and to the student of human fantasy there is nothing new. It has all been experienced before, albeit with slightly different colourations, by millions of others over the centuries. Today's sexual fantasy would have probably taken other forms in history but the task the psyche has to do has always been carried out, whatever the circumstances.

Many pre-school age children fall in love with their opposite-sex parent and wish their same-sex parent would go away (*see* page 41). Little girls often want to marry their father, and little boys express love for their mother. This is a perfectly normal phase of sexual development but it can generate stresses as children have to learn that they can't have mother or father for themselves.

Many studies show that boys and girls are taught their gender roles very early in life. Boys, by and large, end up being active, as girls become comparatively passive. It is clear that well before school age such cultural stereotypes are embedded in a child's psyche. As they start school, boys and girls do not show the gender-related patterns of fantasy found in adult men and women. However, by the age of nine there are clear differences between the fantasies of the sexes. While a boy maintains the fantasies at nine years of age that he had at five, a girl moves from a pattern that mirrors a boy's at five, to one at nine which is much more like that of a woman. Either boys learn about fantasies more slowly (as they learn about many things compared with girls, who tend to catch on faster), or perhaps they are set in more adult-type patterns at the age of five. Only more research will clarify this.

The role of parental fantasies in the formation of their children's fantasies is not known. Numerous studies show that parental attitudes to sex are mirrored by those of their children. There is also good evidence that a person's sexual attitudes are related directly to his or her fantasy life, so clearly there is bound to be some sort of link between the fantasies of parents and their children.

As the years pass, children become involved in the realities of genital sexuality as hormones at puberty trigger an interest in the opposite sex. Now masturbation starts, if it has not already done so, and fantasy takes on a whole new role. This is discussed in more detail on page 39. As adolescence progresses, young people usually begin to interact with the opposite sex. If this interaction is denied them, adolescents create their own sexual realities while awaiting the sexual and emotional maturity that enables them to make something happen in life with a sex partner. Many fantasies originate at this time of high sexual drive, great expectations and low opportunity.

In this brief outline I have tried to show how people come to have fantasies – sexual or otherwise – at all. The problem with understanding the sexual fantasies of adults is that it's very difficult to know, outside the therapy room, how they arrived at any particular fantasy. Which traumatic experience or pleasure, which particular book, person, event or parental attitude gave rise to it? I hope that by reading through some of the most common fantasies and their sources you will be better able to see why you fantasize about certain themes and what these fantasies mean in your life.

DOES EVERYONE FANTASIZE?

Almost certainly, yes. Those who claim not to often have unconscious reasons for repressing their fantasies – usually because they find them somehow unacceptable. A few therapy sessions can often open up the closed areas in the mind and, as if by magic, start the individual fantasizing.

There are, however, many people who are unable to fantasize, simply because they have never trained themselves to be imaginative. As a therapist I'm far more concerned about the first group because the blocked material usually turns out to be central to their problem. But I also see many of the latter group. They dream rarely (or, more accurately, recall few dreams); day-dream hardly at all; aren't very creative; and sometimes think of fantasy as a waste of time or something weirdos do.

With some encouragement and training in imagining scenes, they quickly come to enjoy the fruits of creative fantasy about both sexual and non-sexual subjects. Sometimes this leads to increased creativity at work, at play, in the family and in the bedroom, much to everyone's delight. Reading or hearing about other people's fantasies is sometimes all that is needed to trigger fantasies of their own. Some people I see appear not to know what I'm talking about when the subject is first raised, only to report a few weeks later that they've a rich and exciting fantasy life of their own. It seems that giving permission brings fantasies out from a sort of psychic waiting room.

WHAT USE ARE FANTASIES?

First, fantasies are a way in which previous life events can be dealt with in the present. The perceived reality created in fantasy isn't real, yet it's convincing enough to fool the unconscious in a way that enables the individual to carry on with life without being overwhelmed by the past and its consequences.

In this sense, sexual fantasy is a sort of psychic lifeline to be called upon when things get tough. On occasion a fantasy helps to smother other, less acceptable, fantasy material that the unconscious censor would find difficult to handle. In this way, fantasy can overlay fantasy. But fantasies don't only serve a purpose from the past. They can, like the almost universal fantasy experiences of pregnant women, help people come to terms with anxieties about the future. Pregnancy fantasies, of stillborn or deformed children, for example, have, it seems, a thoroughly healthy purpose in preparing women for the dangers that are intrinsic to this momentous time.

The next most common function of fantasies is, in my opinion, to allow the unconscious to come out to play in an acceptable form. Given that most people have a whole mass of, often contradictory, information lurking in the back of their conscious and unconscious mind on the subject of sex, it is hardly surprising that they sometimes need to let it out within the boundaries that the conscious mind can deal with. The use of symbolism and rigidly controlled scripts helps make this otherwise dangerous task possible. Just what drives the unconscious to create a fantasy at a particular time isn't understood, but my experience suggests that some sort of trigger factor in the present is usually discernible to the aware fantasist or the skilled observer. Such triggers are often extremely subtle. For example, one man went through a period of fantasizing about sadistic themes, but hadn't linked them to his unconscious hostility to his wife since she became pregnant against his wishes. A perfectly well balanced relationship at the conscious level became disturbed by this powerful assertion of her femaleness over his life, and triggered off unrecognized depths of the man's unconscious that he'd hitherto hidden successfully. His hatred of his mother, and his fear of mothers in general, surfaced, much to his amazement.

Not all fantasies have such a momentous origin; quite the opposite. Many people fantasize as a form of waking reverie – they toy with a series of sexual themes. Their minds wander while on a train, waiting for a bus, in bed with their partners – at any time. Some people, doubtless as a result of early childhood experiences, are day-dreamers about non-sexual subjects as well as sexual ones. They readily drop in and out of a dream world they inhabit much of the time. A recent UK study found that the average man thought about sex some 20 times during any one day. My clinical experience shows me that women think about the subject at least as much as men do; clearly sexual reveries and fantasies are extremely frequent in most people's lives. At what point a fleeting thought becomes a true fantasy is open to debate, but the general principle remains true, nonetheless.

FANTASY TO THE RESCUE

Fantasy can be used as a form of auto-hypnosis. Some of my patients practise this expertly at times of stress or boredom. It can be a useful tool to divert panic at the dentist's, the doctor's, or before an exam, for example.

When most people think of sexual fantasies they remember the times when they use such reveries to enhance sexual arousal. This can be when day-dreaming, or during masturbation, foreplay or sexual intercourse. At any of these times a self-created world can make arousal possible, or better than it would otherwise be. This is covered in more detail on page 155.

Fantasy can also help in the absence of a sexual partner. This is most useful for the young, who become sexually active in mind long before Western culture allows them to be so in fact. This deficiency is made good by fantasizing. It is during early and middle adolescence, as events, real and imagined, come to bear on their lives, that most young people learn and re-learn their favourite fantasies. These fantasy patterns are laid down for the future and often remain largely untouched into old age.

The next phase of life when many individuals have no partner is in old age. Today's woman outlives her man by many years on average, and this creates a large pool of older women without partners, who are still sexually active, if only in the mind. For the many millions who can't obtain a partner because there simply aren't enough to go round, fantasy can come to the rescue.

Most people experience a time when their partner is away from home, or is ill or disabled. For them, fantasy has an essential role to play as they seek to make do in a time of sexual famine without recourse to other lovers.

Much research shows that men in particular fantasize because they are dissatisfied with the amount or style of sexual activity they experience in real life. Fantasy can be used in this way to make up for deficiencies in real-life partners. Most men, when asked in surveys, say they want more sex than they get, and many express some dissatisfaction with what their partner does, or doesn't do, in bed. However, there are some people who can never have enough sex. Far from making up for what can be seen as reasonable deficiencies in their love life, they work on the 'more is never enough' principle and have a rich fantasy life with or without masturbation alongside a highly active sex life. It's interesting that there are probably just as many women in this group as there are men, contrary to popular myth.

A CREATIVE SEX AID

Fantasy has another very valuable function as a means of rehearsing or experimenting with an unfamiliar sexual exploit. Many such exploits are difficult, either because they cause embarrassment or because they present practical problems that must be overcome. Fantasizing about the proposed sexual activity gives you the opportunity to explore things in your mind before putting your sexual ego on the line in the bedroom. Sometimes a game that has potential turns out to be a let-down in fantasy, so is left untried. On other occasions anxieties are defused by the fantasy practice run and the actual event goes all the more smoothly as a result. Rehearsal in fantasy can be particularly useful for the young, who are inexperienced and shy.

Some people have conscious sexual needs and desires that are hard, or impossible, to meet with a real-life partner. Some may not even involve a human partner, (*see* pages 125-6). Such people can indulge their fantasies and deal with the underlying unconscious material without recourse to other socialized forms of sexual outlet, such as prostitution. In this way, fantasy is a valuable safety net for millions of individuals who have sexual desires that cannot readily be satisfied in a one-to-one relationship, even if they have one.

Used during sexual intercourse or foreplay, fantasies also enable lovers to enhance the events in hand in a way that permits the best possible arousal. Most people experience occasions when they want to have sex, but are not sufficiently aroused to enjoy it fully. Fantasy can come to the rescue, especially for a man who, for some reason, can't achieve an erection and for whom the addition of fantasy tips the balance from being unable to obtain an erection to having a usable one. His partner, rather than being let down, benefits. How fantasy can help to make sexual failures less likely is discussed on page 151.

In this sense, fantasy is clearly a valuable sex aid in almost any relationship. And unlike commercial sex aids it's tailor-made to suit the user. At one end of the scale such an aid can help a man with a poor erection save the day; at the other, it can be a life-saver for the individual married to someone whom it's impossible, for various reasons, to leave. Individuals in this situation can often lose themselves during intercourse in their fantasy relationship and so make what they have bearable. Among such couples fantasies save families and promote social cohesion. Those who disapprove of the idea of fantasizing within relationships would do well to acknowledge the existence of the many who are trapped in unsuitable relationships, rather than condemn such people for indulging in 'adulterous' thoughts while making love to their partner.

Adultery in the mind is far safer in every way than its real-life equivalent.

However, it is probably preferable to be able to enjoy a full and rich sex life without having to stray, even in the mind. Sex is a whole-person activity involving mind, body and spirit. There can be little doubt that in an ideal world the three should weave together uniquely with those of the partner with whom you make love. To have in mind another place, or fantasy partner, undoubtedly inhibits this total sharing and probably puts a lover at a disadvantage.

I realize that this is a counsel of perfection and that for most people sex can be enhanced in many different ways, but the total absorption in one's partner during true sexual intercourse – that is, sex based on a loving relationship – is one of the features that makes it different from mere copulation.

Making up for deficiencies in a current relationship can take many forms in fantasy, some of which are highly unexpected to those who criticize such activity. For example, I regularly find that people who are incapable of true intimacy in real life can imagine themselves to be so in fantasy. Their real-life problem with intimacy can sometimes be caused by their partner's inability to be intimate with them, but often it is not. If not, such individuals can use fantasy to practise being intimate in a way they want to be deep down, but can't make happen in daily life. I use this sort of modelling, or 'shaping', as it's called, with those I see who want to be more sexual but can't, for whatever reason, make it happen. Encouraging them to fantasize what they want to be like in reality causes them to shape their own fantasies in a way that helps them make new behaviour with a flesh-and-blood partner possible. In this sense fantasy can help transform people from what they are to what they'd like to be.

For some this means becoming a new person only in their fantasy. However, it's possible, and often desirable, to go beyond this to take the transformed sexual being out into the real world and indulge it. I have excellent results with this form of fantasy-shaping and know that any reader can achieve much the same in his or her relationship, with time and open-mindedness.

The majority of people fantasize most often about a current partner (*see* page 53). This is probably highly valuable, because in doing so they invest more in their lovers, and lock their sexual reality into their conscious and unconscious, so enhancing their worth. In modern Western society, which, for reasons of health, is increasingly concerned about promiscuity and one-night stands, anything that increases the esteem in which people hold their partners must be good news. It's well known that brochures are most avidly read by those who have just bought the products they describe. So it is with one-to-one relationships. It's as if human beings need to reassure themselves that what they do is right for them. By fantasizing about a current partner it's possible to keep re-investing the interest from the sexual bank account straight back into the same business. This usually yields the best dividends.

These are some of the more common uses that fantasies have in everyday life. Other, more specific functions are outlined in detail in Part Two.

WHAT ARE THE MOST COMMON FANTASY THEMES?

In Part Two I list more than 40 common fantasies, the subjects of which are varied and numerous. However, it's important to bear in mind, when trying to find out how common or popular any theme is, that people answering questionnaires about their fantasies aren't likely to be totally truthful. Several studies show that people aren't honest when answering questionnaires – even if they are assured of total anonymity. Having studied the world literature on sexual fantasy, I think this may be because most questionnaires are so badly worded that the information can be incomplete and misleading.

Questions such as, 'What is your favourite fantasy?' may appear to be straightforward but aren't. What does 'favourite' mean? Might a favourite fantasy with one partner be different from that with another? What if a favourite fantasy has changed over the last year, let alone over a sexual lifetime? The problems, evidently, are numerous.

Then there is the dilemma of whether the respondent should, when answering a questionnaire, tell the whole truth. This is especially problematical if the fantasy is perceived by its originator as unwholesome, perverted or sinful. Such a fantasy might really be a favourite but may end up being sanitized to avoid possible embarrassment.

At the one extreme I, as a therapist, see quite a few people who claim to have no fantasies at all. When hidden fantasies emerge in therapy, as they usually do, they are often highly guilt-inducing and were obviously repressed by the individual because they couldn't initially be tolerated. In my experience, incest fantasies come high on the list with such people.

With all this in mind I surveyed the world literature, searching every major study over the last 30 years to see what the commonest themes are among males and females. The interesting thing was that the findings of quite well designed studies were so different. Sometimes a subject that was first or second in popularity on one list didn't even appear in the top ten on another. These differences can probably be explained by focusing on the very different populations being studied. As I know to my cost when trying to conduct such studies, one can only get a certain sub-fraction of the population to take part. This has meant that many researchers have used captive audiences, such as university students, as their subjects. This can be misleading as students don't represent the entire adult community. They are highly educated and this is directly related to fantasy frequency (the highly educated fantasize more often). Many of them have not had settled one-to-one relationships and are often at a stage of life when they are experimenting with sex.

One major and highly influential study of the fantasies women use during sexual intercourse, much quoted in the literature, involved mainly Jewish women of the middle and upper classes living in New York City. Again, hardly a broad cross-section of the community.

The trouble is that there's no way to ascertain the truth about such matters as sexual fantasy. One cannot force people to talk about their fantasies, so researchers will always have to accept whatever scant evidence they can discover. As with all other expressions of human sexuality, there is no such thing as a norm in the realms of sexual fantasy; or at least if there is, it's a range and not a point.

The other interesting thing that strikes anyone who has been looking at the subject over some years is that the colouration of sexual fantasies changes with time in any population, and not just because the individuals in that population are getting older. Anyone's fantasies might change over the years, but far more interesting is that men in general are fantasizing about rather different matters today, both in the sexual and non-sexual arenas. As the role of women changes and men's place in the family alters, old fantasies are modified, and new ones created, to take these factors into account.

Let's look at the top fantasies of males and females, as admitted by interviewees in surveys carried out over the last three decades. These lists are the result of combining many studies.

WOMEN'S FAVOURITE REVERIES

Females fantasize most often about their current partner. Reliving a past experience comes next, followed by new love-making positions; oral sex; making love in exotic or romantic places; being forced to have sex; being found irresistible by a man; sex with a new partner; and doing something wicked.

TOP OF THE POPS FOR MEN

Fantasizing about a current partner is also a favourite for males, but giving and receiving oral sex comes second. Sex with two or more women features next, followed by sensual, non-genital love-making; being aggressive or dominant; being made love to; reliving a past experience; and being an onlooker while others have sex.

GENDER DIFFERENCES

One of the most commonly asked questions about fantasy, is 'Do males and females fantasize about the same things?' The short answer is, 'Yes.' Certain themes are more commonly seen in the fantasies of each sex but they are not specific or unique to that sex. Even themes that were, until recently, said to be the sole domain of males, such as fetishes, are now known to be much more widespread among females than was once thought. It's certainly true that as females in Western culture change their behaviour to compete in a largely masculine world, their fantasies are changing. Those who work with fantasy see this almost every day. There is, in my view, no true distinction between the fantasies of the sexes.

Although any sort of generalization about such a complex subject is bound to be fraught with difficulties right from the start, I shall try to summarize the findings of past studies.

By and large males produce more, and more explicit, sexual fantasies than females do. This could be a straight reflection of the fact that female sexuality is more censored by Western culture compared with male sexuality or it could be that many females don't report their romantic fantasies because they think they don't count. Perhaps both apply. Whatever the truth it shouldn't be assumed for a moment that women are poor cousins when it comes to fantasy. Quite the contrary. Women account for more than half of the 100 million porn

---

Many people have fantasies about making love to someone of the same sex, yet they are not gay. Such dreams are almost certainly a way in which people unconsciously make love to the same-sex parts of their personalities.

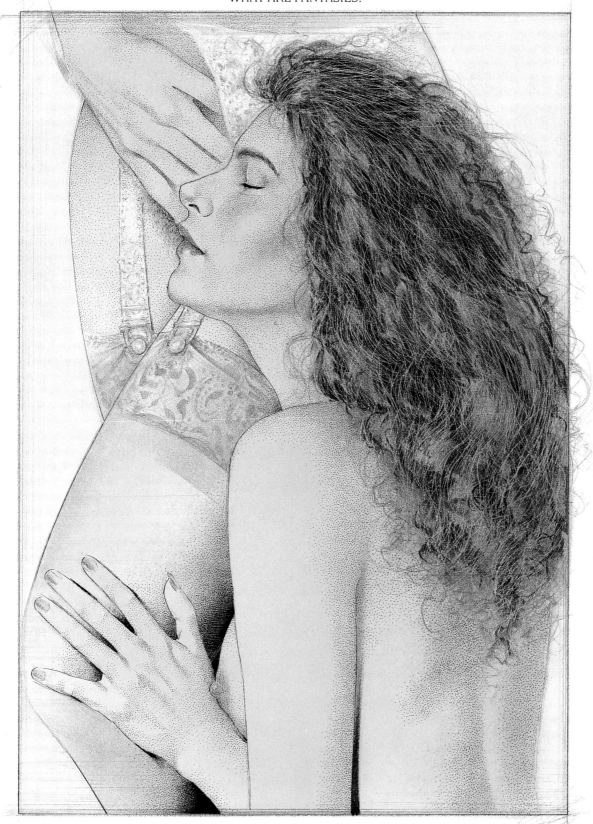

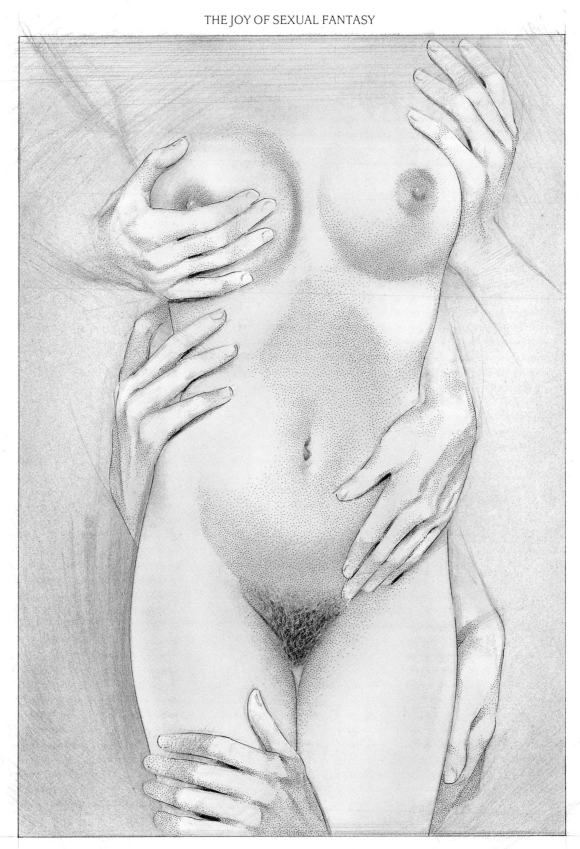

video rentals in the USA and one hard-core porn distributor in Australia claims that one third of all orders are from women. In the USA there is now a porn film company, run by a woman, that creates explicit materials for women.

Males, on balance, say they think about events they have actually experienced whereas females fantasize mainly about things they have never done. This could come about mainly because females tend, more than males, to dwell on imagined experiences in general; or it could mean that women have more unfulfilled wishes than males because they are unable to make desired events happen in their sexual lives. Perhaps more women are guilty and anxious about engaging in sexual behaviour, and so dream about it more than they do it; or it could be that given that both sexes find fantasies of imaginary sexual activities more arousing, men use them less in an effort to delay their single orgasm, and women use them more to produce a bigger and repeated orgasmic response.

After ruling out intimate types of fantasy (passionate kissing, oral sex, romantic sex and masturbating a partner) male fantasies seem to point to a degree of frustration. Men, it seems, fantasize more when their sex life isn't going well, whereas women have more fantasies when things are good. Perhaps women's fantasies are stimulated by, and dependent on, a good sex life; after all, far more of them deal with intimate themes compared with men's fantasies. This is probably linked to the fact that most women can switch off from sex for quite long periods in the absence of a partner, whereas sex for men seems to be a more constant drive that calls for frequent outlets.

The excess of males who are sexually unfulfilled and seeking solace in their fantasy lives might come about because males have, on average, a greater interest in sexual adventure. This may originate as part of the biological imperative for males to impregnate as many females as possible to ensure the survival of their genetic line. The end result of this could be a large number of males complaining about a shortage of sex, or of the sort of adventurous sex they really want. Study after study over the last 40 years has found this to be the commonest complaint men have about sex. However, a woman who feels adventurous as a result of becoming more masculine in her social and sexual orientation in modern society, has no difficulty finding partners to oblige her desires, and so doesn't have many deficiencies to make up for in fantasy.

Women who fantasize a great deal seem to put their fantasies into practice with several different partners, but men are not so lucky. Those with high levels of fantasy are no more successful with women than those without.

Most males and females fantasize about intimate sexual themes, often with their current partner, or a previous one. Exploratory themes, including group sex, promiscuity, partner-swapping and homosexuality are less common in women than men. Men are generally more active in their fantasies than women.

Impersonal fantasies, such as sex with strangers, watching others make love, fetishes, looking at porn or using objects for sexual stimulation are very much less common in women than in men, whereas sado-masochistic fantasies

The many hands of several mystery lovers can transport a woman to ecstasy in her fantasy.

involving whipping, spanking and being forced to have sex are about equally popular with both sexes.

In the light of current discussions regarding the shifting roles of men and women in modern society, some experts claim that the differences in sexual tastes and instincts will become extinct in the near future. My clinical experience and the results of research studies show that this is not happening, at least not with any speed. As judged by what the sexes best enjoy (rather than what they do) both in fact and fantasy, there is no evidence that women have become more like men over the last two generations. Certain themes that were never seen in women – or at least never reported – are now to be found, but overall patterns of female sexual instincts remain very constant. My experience, and that of other clinicians, is that fantasies are hard to change. With considerable motivation and perseverence they can be changed, as is discussed in Part Three. But short-term efforts to change ordinary people's fantasies usually meet with little success. This is perhaps hardly surprising, given the deep-seated unconscious roots of most of them. Repeated exposure to new erotic images and messages in the media will, eventually, change the fantasy life of both sexes, if only a little, but deep down surprisingly little changes with the passage of time.

When both sexes are asked in laboratory experiments to write about or recount their fantasies, male fantasies tend, on balance, to contain more explicit anatomical detail than those of females. Men, in these situations, also write more and in more detail than women do. Perhaps this has something to do with the guilt some women feel about fantasies (see page 32).

My experience is that both sexes write (or recount verbally) their fantasies at much the same length and in the same graphic detail. But I see people of all ages, not just the student populations often studied. As a result, the fantasies reported in Part Two are difficult to 'sex' with any certainty without knowing the gender of the owner. This is in keeping with all my clinical experience, which shows that the sexes are much more alike than different in sexual expression.

As might be expected, people who day-dream most also have the largest number of sexual fantasies. Indeed, according to one study, heavy day-dreamers needed fantasy more than others to become sexually aroused.

Another difference I find when listening to the sexes is that women tend to be more interested in their own feelings and emotional responses during a fantasy, whereas men tend to focus on the effect they're having on the imaginary partner. This fits in with the Western cultural pattern of males making things happen for female lovers, as in romantic fiction.

GAY FANTASIES

The fantasies enjoyed by gay people are remarkably similar in style and content to heterosexual fantasies. Until very recently, the only study that looked at the fantasy life of homosexuals was carried out by Masters and

---

Both the masculine and the feminine components of our personality show themselves, albeit in many disguises, through our fantasies and dreams.

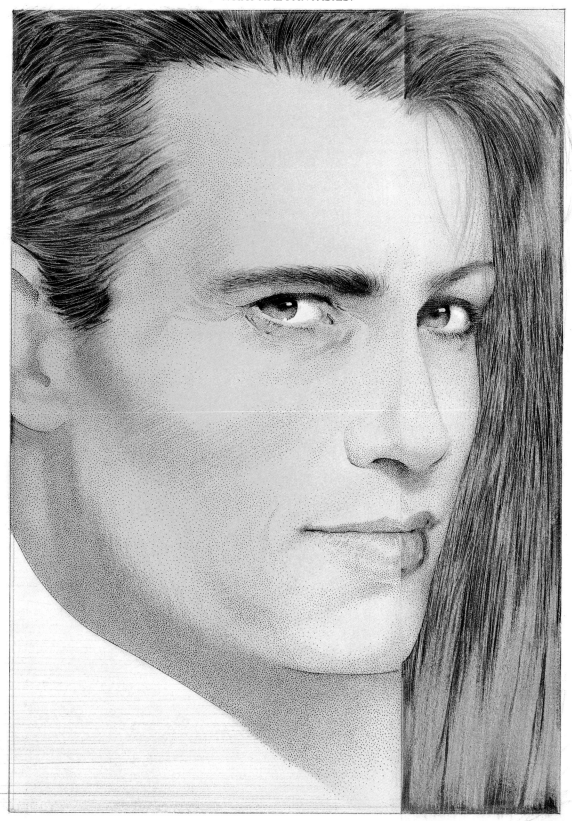

Johnson in 1979. They found that homosexual males had a more active and diverse sexual life than heterosexual males, and that homosexual women had more fantasies than homosexual men. The commonest fantasy in gay men, they found, was thinking about the male body, mainly the penis and buttocks. The other common fantasies were forced sexual encounters (with both men and women), forcing a woman or being forced by a woman to have sex, encounters with unknown men, and observing group sex. The lesbians they studied had fantasies of being forced to have sex, idyllic encounters with a known partner, and sadistic behaviour towards men and women.

Since this study others have found that homosexual fantasies are more similar to those of heterosexuals. In one major US investigation, for example, two of the top three fantasies of homosexual men were the same as those enjoyed by heterosexual men. The only difference, as you'd expect, is that gay men fantasized first and foremost about sex with another man. This study also found that lesbian women didn't have the sex-with-force fantasies Masters and Johnson reported.

As is discussed on page 101, almost everyone has same-sex fantasies at one time or another; and for a few heterosexuals of both sexes such erotic thoughts are their favourites. It should, therefore, come as no surprise to discover that when the fantasies of gay men and women are analyzed, the only really striking difference statistically speaking is that these groups fantasize about sex with someone of their own sex far more often than heterosexuals do.

However, some gay men and women have fantasies about heterosexual intercourse or foreplay, if only from time to time. Why this should be is open to various interpretations. Some lesbian authors claim that it's a way of indulging in what is considered naughty or forbidden sex and that its wickedness is what so appeals. I see it rather differently, though I don't discount this view. To me it's simply a part of the homo-hetero-sexual spectrum that many people inhabit in their fantasy lives. Just as straight people have same-sex fantasies from time to time, gays have heterosexual ones.

When differences between the fantasies of the heterosexual and homosexual communities are found, gay fantasies seem in the main to relate more to anatomical and mechanical sexual matters than do fantasies from matched heterosexuals. This means that there tend to be more mentions of specific parts of the body, anal sex, and sado-masochistic activities. However, one large study found that romantic fantasies are by far the most common in gay men.

Like heterosexuals, gay people fantasize not so much about specific, rigidly laid-down subjects, as about a range of sexual activities. The choice of activity as a subject of fantasy depends on how an individual feels at the time.

Most homosexual men and women are happy to remain gay, but a few want to change their orientation and become straight. Many studies have found that homosexual people can change sexual preference to some extent, by modifying their fantasies.

FANTASY AND GUILT

Sex in Western Judaeo-Christian culture is a subject riddled with guilt. Around the time that the Old Testament was written, sex was controlled and regulated by the establishment, as a small tribe of ancient Jews tried to battle for survival against considerable odds. As a result, their attitudes to sexuality were different in many respects from those of most other contemporary peoples around the world, particularly those of the sexually sophisticated Orient.

Although Jesus said very little about sexuality, and was certainly not negative on the matter, many of His followers used Christian 'churchianity' as a way of dealing with their personal dogmas, with the result that sex was degraded. The damage done by the early Christian fathers is hard to over-estimate; and in many conscious and unconscious ways their legacy lives on today.

With this sex-negative culture as a backdrop, it's difficult to escape the fact that many people feel guilty about their erotic fantasies. Research shows that this is especially true of women. Judaeo-Christian culture suppresses the sexuality of women much more than that of men and has the ability to make women feel guilty about sex on the slightest pretext. While it's a fact that this level of sex guilt is lower than it was a generation or two ago, clinicians like me never cease to be amazed at how little things have in fact changed. At the deeply unconscious level many more women of all ages are negative about sex or feel guilty or anxious about it than most people would think possible.

It's still considered disgraceful for a woman to be seen as sexually pushy, although attitudes are slowly changing. It isn't acceptable for women to procure their own seduction, though more of them take the lead in and out of bed. Even many of those who do so, and I suggest that they are still in the minority, tell me they really want the man to take charge most of the time.

What ensues when a man conducts the sexual orchestra is that he takes responsibility for the woman's sexual pleasure, thereby exonerating her from the guilt she feels either consciously or unconsciously at being overtly sexual. 'He did it to me, the dirty devil,' is the sort of message. My life as a sexual and marital therapist is daily sprinkled with such thoughts and even overt statements. I see this even among young, supposedly streetwise women who claim, and indeed appear, to be liberated.

THE SHADOW OF GUILT

With all of this as a background, it's hardly surprising that many more women than men claim not to fantasize. If women do admit to fantasizing, they often sanitize their erotic reveries to make them acceptable to their unconscious censor. Naturally, some men also feel guilty about sex, for the same reasons as women. Sex guilt is certainly not the preserve of females.

What exactly is guilt in this context? It's the expectancy that there will be some sort of self-induced punishment for violating the standards of culturally accepted sexuality. It is possible to measure sex guilt levels; and when this is done it becomes evident that those who are very guilty think less about sex, do less about it and fantasize less about it. They also report more stress, guilt and embarrassment after being exposed to sexual stimuli.

Various studies have looked at sex guilt. Although the results of some of the early ones suggested that most females experience high levels of sexual arousal in spite of their guilt, others have found that those women with low sex guilt are most easily aroused.

Most recent studies find that females with low sex guilt have more fantasies, and that these fantasies are more detailed, longer and more varied in subject matter, than those of women with high levels of guilt about sex. Substantially more females with high levels of guilt about sex have fantasies about being dominated by a male and being irresistible to men than women with low levels of guilt. High-sex-guilt women tend to have more fantasies about imaginary or faceless lovers; low-sex-guilt women tend to fantasize about real people. As there's no difference in the levels of arousal reported by the favourite fantasies of either group, it is clear such reveries do the job. Research shows that whatever the level of sex guilt it's possible, given a large enough stimulus, for even a very guilty individual to become aroused.

Several research studies, and my clinical experience, suggest that high-sex-guilt women experience their fantasies less vividly and remember them less well than their low-sex-guilt sisters do. As I explain on page 25, it's extremely hard to interpret what people report of their fantasies. Once the concept of sex guilt is studied, it's easy to see how it can drastically modify what any individual will report. Negative attitudes to sex, however unconscious, produce negatively toned fantasies and less sexual arousal. Research has found that those who claim to be religious have significantly fewer and less rich and less explicit fantasies, than non-religious people.

It is consistently found that females have more obviously romantic fantasies than males do. I suspect that this has much to do with guilt reduction. In a romantic fantasy the man takes the lead and absolves the woman from any associated guilt, either at the time or afterwards. Some people say that it isn't the act of masturbation itself that makes them feel guilty, but the associated fantasies. This response applies to both sexes, but more to women.

By and large it's fair to say that as people of either sex become more sexually experienced they encounter less guilt about sex. With this in mind, it's hardly surprising to find that virgins of either sex fantasize less often and less vividly than sexually experienced people do. In one study sexual experience was the best predictor of frequency of fantasizing. Among males, experience was the best predictor of explicitness and frequency of fantasizing. The best possible predictor of fantasy length in this research was sex guilt, for both sexes.

I've discussed guilt at length because so many people, women particularly, are dogged by it. It prevents them fantasizing about subjects that would otherwise arouse them greatly; spoils their arousal when they do use them; and makes them feel bad afterwards. I look on page 151 at a simple way of overcoming guilt feelings, although I realize that there will always be some individuals whose guilt cannot be dealt with in this DIY way. For them, professional help can often yield excellent results.

Guilt is often at the heart of the problem when someone tells me they don't fantasize. They are, in fact, fantasizing, but their unconscious censor interrupts the fantasy and shuts it out of their conscious mind before it can take hold. I often find that simply reading a book about the fantasies of others, or talking the subject over with me for a few hours, opens the door, and gives the unconscious censor permission to go off duty while they allow their fantasies to come to the fore.

LOVING TO DEATH

A fascinating postscript to the subject of guilt and fantasy is the connection between death anxiety and sexual fantasies. Sex and the fear of death are closely interlinked in the unconscious, and sometimes even in the conscious. The French have called orgasm *le petit mort* – the little death. A few women actually lose consciousness when having an exceptionally powerful orgasm; and I find my patients fascinated by the connection between these two taboo subjects.

Some women who are unable to have orgasms tell me that they fear they might die if they were to lose control sufficiently to have one. Others talk of a symbolic 'dying' in sex, to be 'resurrected' afterwards to create new life in some mystical sense, and I find this a perfectly acceptable concept and very helpful to many. Sex is, after all, a restorative experience for many people. Some say they feel truly alive when in a good sexual relationship, and somehow dead when they're not.

As would be expected, the psychoanalytical giants have had their say on the matter of sex and death. It is generally claimed that sex is at one and the same time the most intense human pleasure and the most pervasive human anxiety. Freud and Rollo May made much of the link between sex and death, and one analyst claimed that sex is fused with expectations of injury and anxiety.

Death anxiety can be measured quite accurately, using highly specialized questionnaires. It's usually found that the link between death and sexuality is more prevalent among women than among men. Perhaps this comes about as a result of women's association with death in the process of creating new life. Until the last century death in childbirth was a real possibility for many women. As I talk about this with women today, many tell me of a sort of 'dying' during a normal labour, almost as if they had to die in some way. They then say they felt reborn – as a different person – with the baby.

A major study found that those people who had high or low death anxiety had more sexual fantasies than those who had only moderate death anxiety. It has been suggested that a high level of sexual fantasy in an individual acts to conceal the fear of death. This study tended to back up these findings. Perhaps those who are aware of death and even anxious about it focus on the transitory nature of life and so go for pleasures of the moment, abandoning themselves to sexual fantasy. Perhaps a concern with death makes such people more aware of the impulses of the body, which in turn produces more fantasies. Certainly those who have a high level of concern with death are found to have a high level of interest in fantasy, day-dreams and internal bodily sensations.

Individuals who are anxious about death may be trying, unconsciously, to neutralize their high levels of fantasy by coupling them with high levels of punishment in the form of death. There is no evidence of this, but in Western culture there is a considerable association between death, punishment and sex. Many women I talk to believe that if they do something they see as naughty or sinful, they will somehow be punished. This ostensibly wicked act may be something as ordinary as really enjoying sex, or taking the lead in bed.

'Now that I have had the pleasure, I should expect the pain' is a classic, unconscious, Judaeo-Christian notion regarding sexuality. Some people tell me that even having a highly arousing sexual fantasy makes them feel that some sort of divine retribution in the form of a thunderbolt or similar punishment will be visited upon them. They then list adverse events and episodes in everyday life as evidence of such punishable behaviour.

Although I can deal only briefly with this fascinating connection between death and sex, in fantasy the two often come together in a way that might not always be apparent. I hope the subject has provided some food for thought.

DO PERVERTED FANTASIES MAKE ME A PERVERT?

The answer is almost certainly, no. Most people's idea of a perversion, ie 'something you want to do that I don't like', is clearly much too limited a way of viewing life in general and a partner's sexuality in particular. I believe that in a truly loving and committed relationship there is no such thing as a perversion. If people can accept their lovers as they are, in true unconditional love, whatever they declare about themselves will be accepted. However, as I see in my practice, just because someone finds a sexual preference hard to take, the partner who suggests it isn't necessarily wrong, odd or perverted. Whatever is revealed has to be looked at in the context of social norms, the norms for the relationship, and what can be coped with at any one time. Fantasies of having sex with little girls, for example, would be seen as socially unacceptable, so it would be wrong to indulge such a preference in a partner. But where to draw the line when matters are less clear-cut depends on the individual couple.

FEAR AND FASCINATION

There will always be differences when it comes to matters of sexual taste. And no-one should feel obliged to endure a partner's sexual fantasies if they are at odds with one's own sexuality. But by rejecting the 'perverted' fantasy it's hard to avoid being seen as rejecting the individual who entertains it. After all, it's highly likely that a person chooses a partner because he or she is attracted to the personality capable of having such fantasies. A woman I saw recently complained that her man was a pervert because she was expected to listen to his fantasy about tying her up to have sex. She, an ardent feminist, found this idea abhorrent. The thought of being so degraded was, to her, quite horrific and she couldn't imagine how she'd come to marry such an oddball. It rang warning bells from her childhood, reminding her of a violent, overbearing father who used to give her mother a hard time.

After much reflection and deeper therapeutic work over some weeks I encouraged her to become less certain about how right she was and how evil her husband's fantasy wishes were. Once we obtained a degree of acceptance and tolerance I suggested tentatively that they might, one day, try to act out in a highly symbolic way the fantasy she'd found so disgusting. This suggestion brought forth an outpouring of invective about how men (including me) have to dominate and use women. But to her enormous credit she did eventually go along with my suggestion, after a few drinks. The result was stunning. She became so aroused she couldn't believe it; and at first she didn't want to. She reported having multiple orgasms for the first time ever.

This, understandably, led to much soul-searching on this woman's part. It soon became obvious to her that she had somehow known, unconsciously, that she and her man were well matched in this regard. Deep down she wanted to be dominated and he had the perfectly conscious need to behave in this way toward her. Clearly, they had unconsciously chosen one another to answer their mutual needs. My patient's choice of partner clearly reflects her relationship with her father: she had chosen to marry a similar type of man. This situation is very common indeed, but may not be at all obvious, unless the partners dig deep into their unconscious.

Even the simplest of tying-up games revealed these hidden aspects of their relationship, and my patient's internal battle about men being domineering brutes, a conflict consciously present since her teens, began to abate. Although at first her body seemed, in her words, 'to be taking (her) over' she soon came to see that it was telling her something very real about herself.

Needless to say, her husband was thrilled and the pair enriched their lives together in many ways, both in and out of bed, as a result. Her giving in to her unconscious desires did not, as she'd feared, lead to a cascade of events forcing her man to became a chauvinist pig; quite the contrary. He became more relaxed about her desire to express her feminist ideas, and once he understood that many of them came from the same origins as her fear of his so-called perversion, he was able to help her express them in more positive and creative ways. They came to understand her parents' relationship better: and the husband's 'sadistic' tendencies became limited to their agreed bedroom games rather than spilling over into everyday life as had previously been the case.

Given that so many fantasies yield what could be termed perverted or odd material, interactions of this sort become rather important. Even when acting out a fantasy is impossible, as it is for many couples, considerable insights can be obtained into a partner's personality. With loving acceptance and sharing, this knowledge can be put to excellent use outside the bedroom, in family life, at work, at play, and during sex.

The acting out of so-called deviant fantasies takes some careful handling if you're trying it out without professional guidance. Always go for less than you think you'd like on the grounds that it's always easier to go forward slowly than to mess things up by going too far. Try symbolic enactments rather than a full-frontal attack on the subject matter in hand. For example, anal sex can be fantasized about while making love vaginally in a rear-entry position; tying-up games can be done with a necktie or a silk scarf rather than ropes; and black stockings and high-heeled shoes make a good start for prostitute fantasies. As you become braver and feel safer you can turn up the heat by including more realism, both with props and actions. Even what at first appear quite deviant fantasies can, with this gentle and sensitive approach, be successfully handled until the whole fantasy can be acted out and the excitement enhanced by calling on your imagination.

If you're ever worried that your partner cannot keep within the boundaries you set and the situation appears to be getting out of control, stop and step back from your games. There's a fine line between what one person finds a turn-on and the other a turn-off. In many such adventures reading real and unconsciously mediated turn-offs can be very difficult, even for a professional like me, who deals with them all day. The woman I quoted above is a case in point. Had her protestations been taken at face value she would never have discovered what she did and her relationship would have been much the poorer for it. It took courage and faith on her part to alter the pattern of a lifetime.

But deviant fantasies don't have to be dealt with only in the context of acting them out. Many people would find such behaviour unacceptable, perhaps even threatening. Some women, in particular, find that their men's oddball fantasies make them alarmed about the person they've become involved with. A word of warning: the man who, after only a few dates, reveals an odd fantasy should be regarded with considerable suspicion unless you know him well and can trust him. Women are at serious risk from men they hardly know who seem to make unusual sexual demands either in fact or fantasy. If in doubt, get out.

DANGEROUS FANTASIES

Even if deviant fantasies are sometimes acceptable (albeit in a modified form) as an addition to a couple's sexual repertoire, there will always be relationships in which one partner or the other finds the whole idea unacceptable and will, as a result, want to rid the partner of the fantasy material that is hard to cope with. Alas, there's no way a person can change his or her partner's deviant fantasies by wishing, or even bullying, them away. Just as two lovers can help enrich a deviant fantasy and feed it to their hearts' delight, so the opposite can be made to work if both partners want it to.

Extinguishing a problem fantasy that gets in the way of a happy sexual relationship starts with an honest desire to take on the task. Let's say, for example, that a man has fantasies about homosexual activity and these get in the way of love-making with his wife. By introducing more heterosexual fantasy material, starting near the point of orgasm and, working backward to the start of the fantasy, on successive occasions, encouraging results can often be achieved.

Start off by changing the homosexual fantasy to a heterosexual one about your partner as you make love, right at the moment of ejaculation. The brain quickly starts to associate the pleasures of orgasm with sexual intercourse with your partner, and with your thoughts about making love with your partner. More and more heterosexual detail can now be included at each love-making session until eventually the whole fantasy is heterosexual, alongside a real heterosexual encounter. A man who persists with this, helped by his partner, can often completely extinguish what he feels is an undesirable fantasy over a period of some weeks. From time to time the old fantasy might return, particularly at times of stress, but it can now be seen for what it is – a rarity – rather than a troublesome recurrent theme.

In this way loving partners can act as highly effective sex therapists for one another, especially if they can increase arousal by suggesting other, more stimulating fantasy themes to take the place of the old ones.

Dealing with your own deviant fantasies, then, can be tricky. First, you have to come to terms with them in your mind, and this can be difficult enough, but I often find that things work out best if they're shared with a partner. Just airing the subject can work wonders, because being accepted along with your odd desires can make you feel secure enough to explore them further. Finding that your partner has parallel or reciprocal fantasies can create a sense of closeness and intimacy that's hard to equal. More on how to share fantasies can be found on page 153.

Odd fantasies may be an indicator of true sexual deviancy, the sort that could land the person who has them in trouble with the law, a partner, or both. If this is so, it's wise to seek professional help sooner rather than later, because such fantasies feed on themselves and become more deeply entrenched as the years go by, perhaps even resulting in a desire to do something about them outside the relationship. It's worth bearing in mind that many people don't have a trusting one-to-one relationship, and that some have no relationship at all. For such individuals an empathic, sensitive professional can provide alternatives to living with permanent guilt, shame and fear.

For the vast majority of people, deviant fantasies remain just that: fantasies. They don't act them out either within their relationships or outside them. But for many people some sort of actualization of their deviant needs becomes desirable or, rather, unstoppable, if only from time to time. Such people then seek sex outside their one-to-one relationship to fill the gap in a way that doesn't jeopardize their main partnership. The vast pornography industry caters to this need in men and, increasingly, in women. This is a sort of half-way house between thinking about it and doing something about it, and as such serves a widespread social need.

Fantasies that appear deviant won't go away. They are a part of the individual's sexuality and have to be dealt with somehow. Whether this occurs inside or outside a relationship, in fact or fantasy, will be up to the people involved.

FANTASY AND MASTURBATION

It's impossible to discuss erotic fantasy without looking at masturbation. Self-induced erotic pleasures start very early in life. In the first few weeks of life a baby learns that his or her mouth is full of excitement, and it's clear to any mother who has watched her breast-feeding baby that the child obtains far more than milk from the experience. The blissful expression on the face, the total joy, perhaps even obvious signs of genital arousal are all apparent.

As I take adults through this stage of their psychosexual development in regression sessions they often become noticeably aroused, many of them making the conscious link between oral pleasure and genital eroticism for the very first time in their lives. The results that accrue from this sort of insight and experience can be formidable. Foodies, compulsive drinkers, heavy smokers and other orally-fixated individuals come to see their oral tendencies for what they are. Once addressed in the conscious mind, oral cravings that plague adult life become easier to deal with.

In the next stage of psychosexual development a baby discovers that a bowel movement produces agreeable sensations and, in a similar way to the mouth, this area of the anatomy becomes eroticized. The sexuality of a baby or a very young child is said to be polymorphous, in that almost anything can be experienced as erotic. Some of this lingers on into the child's fantasy life and well into adulthood. This helps explain how almost anything can be eroticized

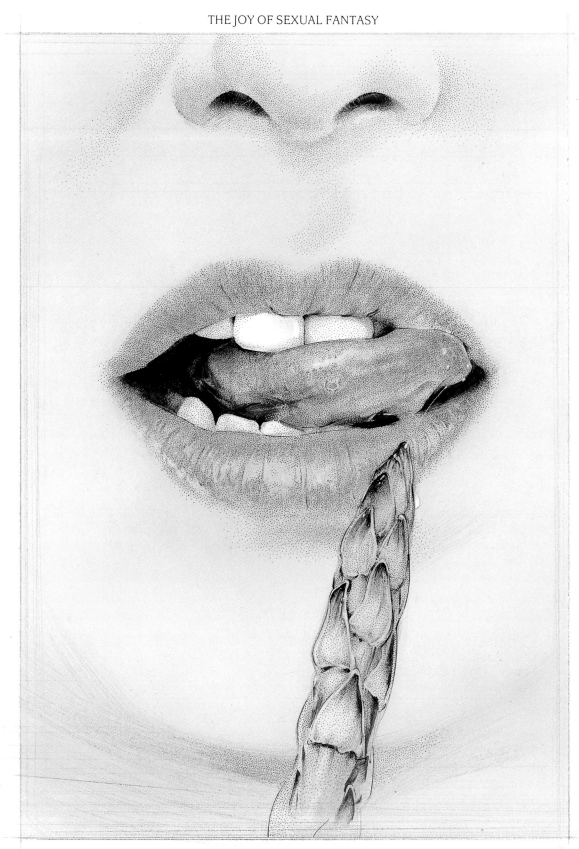

in adult life and why there are so many fantasy themes, many of which at first appear far from erotic to those individuals who have no interest in them.

Both these types of link are accompanied by fantasies that are both consciously acknowledged and unconsciously experienced. Such fantasies come to form the foundations for the deep-seated fantasies of later life.

The next stage of a child's psychosexual development involves feelings toward his or her parent of the opposite sex. At this stage the genitals become a recognized pleasure site and the little child plays with them while fantasizing. Between the ages of three and five some of these fantasies involve the opposite-sex parent. At this stage of development many boys say they want to marry mother, and girls want mother to go away to leave the ground free for them to be alone with father. Old fantasies that were associated with genital arousal in infancy now resurface and the child starts to build in active physical pleasuring alongside the fantasy. But this linking of desire for the opposite-sex parent and genital pleasure brings delight tinged with guilt. Fear of punishment by the same-sex parent is high on the agenda, threatening to turn the most profound love affair to date (that with a parent) into a nightmare. Because of this, such Oedipal fantasies – as they're called – are among the most heavily repressed and the least often revealed in questionnaire studies. Repressed Oedipal fantasies don't, however, go away. They apear in many disguised forms during nocturnal dreams, conscious day-dreams and erotic fantasies.

The physical manifestations of masturbation – erotic self-stimulation – can masquerade in children as nail-biting, thumb- or finger-sucking or obsessively playing with objects. Sometimes an oral erotic pleasure is all too obvious, which is probably why such habits are so vigorously discouraged by adults. But who knows what's going on in the child's mind? Many children, or, in later life, adults, claim that their mind is blank while masturbating. This can't be true. It's a contradiction in terms to say that during conscious waking life the mind is ever truly without content. What the mind's eye sees as a blank screen is as much a fantasy as the perception that it is filled with images.

The absence of fantasy during masturbation almost certainly represents some kind of defensive mechanism which prevents the individual seeing what's on the screen. This becomes clear when practitioners use hypnosis or regression techniques of various kinds to remove even quite deep unconscious masks from the screen and enable the individual to see what was always there.

Many people, when asked about masturbation, claim that it starts at puberty. Most people do indeed have a considerable increase in sexual drive at this time of life and it's true that most children's fantasy life starts to grow very fast at this phase of their sexual development. Nevertheless, about a third of all females I see report that they can't remember a time when they've not masturbated – from babyhood. And it's perfectly clear to any observant parent that babies and young children stimulate their genitals in various direct and indirect ways to produce orgasms or high levels of sexual arousal.

Eating can be highly erotic, especially as a part of love-making. The symbolism of the woman's mouth (vagina) with parted lips (labia) and the approaching phallus is indisputable.

Most children learn early on in life to be secretive about their masturbation and many, girls especially, develop covert ways of achieving high levels of sexual arousal without anyone being aware of it. This is apparent in the many women I see with orgasm problems. They usually masturbate in indirect ways that involve little or no contact with the genitals, but it's certainly masturbation in every sense of the word – and they know it, however unconsciously.

This makes assessing the prevalence of masturbation in females very difficult. Many women I see claim not to masturbate and not to have fantasies. Yet on even quite superficial questioning it becomes clear that both are untrue. I'm sure that about nine out of ten females, and a slightly higher number of males, masturbate. Indirect stimulation methods are rare in males, but not at all uncommon in females, but all this proves is how much more modern culture suppresses the open expression of sexuality in females.

Masturbation and fantasy are inextricably interlinked. Although it's foolish to claim that the former can't take place without the latter, I'm sure that for the vast majority of people the two go together like ham and eggs. Youngsters learning about their sexuality are often surprised and even embarrassed by the pressing nature of their fantasies in early adolescence. What was previously unthinkable or forbidden becomes not only compelling but highly exciting and this, combined with the physical rewards of sexual release, connects the mind with the body in a way that creates a masturbation 'script' that can last a lifetime, albeit perhaps in thinly veiled disguises.

Most people use fantasy when they masturbate. This brings one major

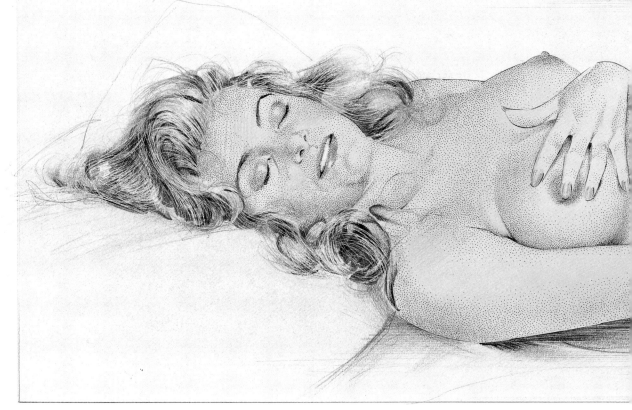

Fantasy is an ideal time to try out new love positions before making them real with a lover.

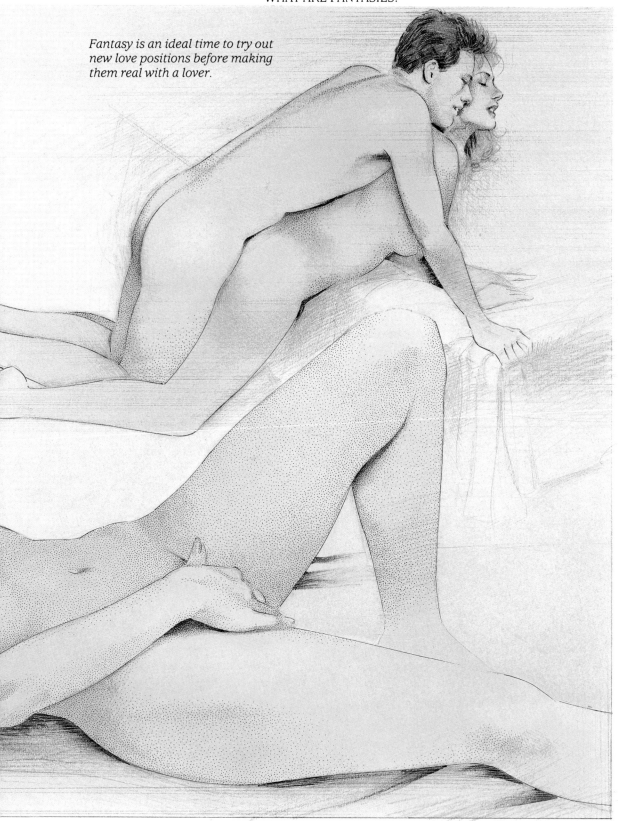

advantage: very high levels of arousal; and one major disadvantage: a sense of guilt. As I have pointed out, some people are guilty about masturbation, not because of the act itself, which they both consciously and unconsciously enjoy and cope with, but rather because of the accompanying fantasies.

Masturbation is to sexual intercourse as talking is to debating, so I see it as an important tool in the sexual life of everyone, whether it's consciously acknowledged or not. This makes fantasy one of the most important areas of human sexuality because it colours all sexual dealings through a lifetime.

Fantasy isn't, of course, necessary for arousal to occur. Many people can achieve very high levels of arousal by being stimulated physically without any fantasy at all. What fantasy does is heighten excitement and make arousal possible, when otherwise it might not be.

Another, less obvious function of fantasy during masturbation is that it helps people play various parts of their character against one another. A patient of mine started to fantasize about looking on while two women made love. At first he became a little concerned that he might, in his words, 'be getting into lesbian fantasies', but on quite superficial scrutiny of the current state of his therapy it became clear that he was coming to terms, in his unconscious, with the feminine parts of his personality which hitherto had been making him guilty and anxious. Fantasies such as these can deal with, and synthesize, the many different and changing parts of an individual's personality. This makes any interpretation of fantasies a difficult process because things may not be what they seem at first.

FANTASY AND SEXUAL EXCITEMENT

Reading the medical and lay literature about fantasies, you could be forgiven for believing that the link between excitement and fantasy is almost never mentioned. This comes about because sexual excitement is rarely the subject of serious research and is largely ignored by analysts, sexologists, and therapists.

The main problem is that the notion of sexual excitement is so imprecise; even defining the phrase is hard enough. Perhaps the best way to think of it is to see excitement as a state of expectancy in which an anticipation of danger alternates with an equal expectation of the avoidance of danger. In the case of sex, danger is replaced by pleasure. However, for a surprisingly great number of people, pleasure paradoxically represents a sort of danger. Many people are pleasure haters and avoiders, especially when the pleasure involves sex. Sex, it has been said, is the greatest source of anxiety in human beings and, as such, is acknowledged by some, consciously and unconsciously, as positively dangerous. In some ways, excitement is a mental state produced by fantasy, which in turn is based on past experience reinvented or remembered to serve a current need.

Various types of excitement are generated by various fantasy styles. The excitement of the cross-dresser is different from the non-genital body excitement of a woman imagining a sadistic attack, for example. They are also rather different physiologically; and the background events that produce them are unique to any individual.

But if excitement is difficult or almost impossible to define or measure, it's even harder to work out why one individual is excited by, say, silk stockings, another by a woman with large buttocks, and yet another by men with slim thighs. Why do feet excite one man but not another? Why do hairy men attract some women and not others?

One of the reasons why all this is fraught with problems for the academic is that fantasy, unlike so many other areas of the human psyche, flourishes on secrecy, disguise, repression, guilt and shame. It has precious little to do with good, honest lust. As soon as a fantasy is exposed to scientific scrutiny, it can interfere with that other elusive flower in the sexual garden – excitement.

What is known is that fantasy helps create excitement, but it appears from clinical experience that several factors are at the heart of all fantasies, although not usually all at once. The main psychological themes are: hostility; mystery; risk; illusion; revenge; a reversal of trauma or frustration to triumph; and some form of dehumanization. How all of these are variously acted out in fantasy is examined in Part Two.

Hostility features in many fantasies of both sexes. At first this seems odd, but because children can't defend themselves from attackers (usually their parents) in real life, they're comforted by being able to do so in day-dream fantasies. This preserves a child's sense of self, restores the balance of power, preserves erotic capacity, and might even be a way of seeking revenge. In this way the child deals with the anger and hostility of others by internalizing it, making it safe, and – perhaps – by overlaying it with rewards in the form of sexual sensations and emotions.

Many games and stories that are evergreen favourites in childhood involve considerable levels of hostility. Whenever I discuss hostile, sadistic fantasies with my patients, I'm frequently reminded of the hostile, sadistic material my own children are, and have been, exposed to in the form of 'Tom and Jerry' cartoons, fairy tales and much other highly popular fiction written for children.

It's easy to see how the excitement of being angry, hostile or vengeful now becomes mixed up with erotic sensations in the mind and body and how the whole blend can be triggered at any point in the circuit. Some people affected in such ways can become sexually aroused only when angry; feel hostile when aroused; cannot separate anger from arousal, or vice versa; or become aroused (or hotly deny their sexuality) when issues of power are raised. It is evident that aggression increases sexual arousal in controlled experiments (*see* page 97), and many couples admit that they make love most passionately after a blazing fight or argument.

It's interesting to bear in mind that humour, like sexual excitement, is hostility subdued and made socially tolerable. The power of humour speaks for itself. Indeed, there are many areas of life that can safely be dealt with only humorously or in fantasy.

WHEN DO PEOPLE FANTASIZE MOST?

Many studies have addressed this question with different results, but overall the order of frequency turns out to be: during day-dreaming, masturbation, and then sexual intercourse.

Many people think about sex, or have a full-blown sexual fantasy, several times a day. In comparison they might masturbate only once every few days, and have sex with about the same frequency. As with all areas of sexuality there are no norms, only rages.

Those who feel they have a satisfactory sex life have more sexual intercourse more frequently, but no direct link is found between fantasy and sexual satisfaction. Those who are satisfied and those who are not seem to enjoy fantasies on similar themes and with much the same content, according to research, but those who are most satisfied with their sex life are more likely to fantasize about their partners. Fantasies have been found to help many married women achieve arousal and orgasm during sexual intercourse, irrespective of their current level of sexual satisfaction.

But the matter of sexual satisfaction is too large and unwieldy to be considered in detail in this book; it's complex enough within any one couple. In one study 63 per cent of the women and 40 per cent of the men in 'happy' marriages were found to have sexual dysfunctions. In another study, sex was the number one area of conflict in 50 'very happily married' couples and eighth or ninth in importance in 50 'very unhappily married' couples.

It's also important to draw distinctions between sexual satisfaction and marital satisfaction. A large number of people who report sexual dissatisfaction say they're happily married. But the very same sexual dysfunction can mean different things to different couples. Many people experience some sort of dissatisfaction, yet don't make much of it, or may even ignore it.

Sexual dysfunctions also have different types of impact on men and women. In general, women put more stress on the importance of the distant past, on non-sexual themes and on how they feel, whereas men tend to emphasize imagery and fantasy more than do women. Sexual and emotional responses to first sexual intercourse feature more in the thoughts and fantasies of women than of men, and when one looks at fantasies in marriages it's clear that a woman's relationship with her mother (both past and present) has much more bearing on her life than does her relationship with her man. I always tell such men that they have two women in their beds when making love with their partners, and they all know exactly what I mean.

Happily married women tend to have a more varied fantasy life than their unhappy sisters do. Happy wives and faithful wives are less likely to fantasize about an imaginary lover or about being a different, more sexy woman. It appears that happily married women are satisfied with themselves as well as their husbands. Studies have also found that orgasmic women are less likely to fantasize about a previous sexual experience than women who can't achieve orgasm.

It's interesting to point out here just how inaccurate women are at assessing their sexual arousal on any occasion. It is my clinical experience that many women, especially those who have sexual problems, have trouble deciding whether or not they're aroused. Even when there's good evidence to suggest that they are aroused, their mind tells them they're not. This cut-off at the neck is undoubtedly governed by the unconscious; a fact which can readily be demonstrated as matters improve after only a few weeks in therapy.

Several studies involving the measurement of vaginal blood flow and the production of vaginal wetness have found that many women can't link what their mind senses with what their body is experiencing. It is interesting that some women are better at making these correlations at certain times of the month than at others. Most women find they're better at gauging their real level of sexual arousal when the fantasy they use is their own – as opposed to one supplied by a researcher. Also, many women seem better able to tell how aroused they are when attending to internal cues, as opposed to outside stimuli. In fact, it's often found that the more a woman is tuned into an external stimulus of some kind, the less she's able to attend to internal cues and thus to her degree of sexual arousal.

A woman who doesn't rate a stimulus as arousing is less likely to be aware of her genital responses. One study which involved playing tapes of romantic fiction to women led to most of the subjects saying they weren't aroused, even though all the scientific measurements showed they were. Conversely, if a woman expects to be aroused she says she is, even though the measurements of her arousal show she isn't.

I have talked about this in some detail, not just because I find women are fascinated by it, but because it's helpful to the understanding of excitement and arousal under the influence of fantasy. Men have an easily visible 'feedback device': the penis. This enables them to monitor their arousal in various situations. The value of this in sexual learning is clear. It's also easy for a man or his partner to learn which fantasies are of most value to him.

On the other hand, unless they're familiar with the degree of their vaginal wetness (the equivalent of male erection), women have no such easy gauge, and are thus less likely to know how aroused they are. With experience, any woman can learn to become just as accurate at assessing her arousal as any man, but this takes time and makes it all the more difficult to know how useful a fantasy is. A woman may find a fantasy really sexy and yet be quite dry. This can lead to misunderstandings in a relationship because, although she may feel randy, her man feels her vagina, finds she's dry and concludes she's not ready to receive him. The reverse can also occur.

Women, like men, can generate full genital responses in the absence of external arousing stimuli and it's interesting that those women who fantasize most can generate the highest genital response levels. The best way for a woman to obtain her highest level of arousal is for her not only to fantasize during masturbation, but to masturbate, having acquired the habit of fantasizing while masturbating. I spend a great deal of time clinically helping and encouraging women to build up their sexual fantasy life as a part of bringing their sex life under their personal control. Such women end up being much more satisfied, both in and out of bed, than their sisters who leave their sexual arousal to their partners and take little or no responsibility for it.

When women such as these start their 'training', I encourage them to think very specifically of insertion, vaginal containment, vaginal sensations, the thrusting of the penis, how their vaginas feel when stimulated with fingers, and other sensations. If a fantasy is constructed with detailed scenes that focus on these matters, even a woman who finds orgasm difficult to achieve can start to gain orgasmic control. The rewards of masturbation enhance all this further and it's usually not long before the whole mixture can be incorporated into her sex life. In this way, many women become able to experience an orgasm during sexual intercourse for the first time. I find the most orgasmic women in such therapy mix both romantic and frankly erotic fantasies.

When considering male sexual arousal it's always said that pictorial material (or at least a visual stimulus) is most effective. Certainly, it's true that most males learn first about female anatomy from pictures. When studies are done, colour slides, spoken text, written text, film and fantasy all produce a build-up of sexual arousal. Once this is achieved, though, the highest level of physiological response is produced by film, and the lowest by fantasy.

Males, it seems, respond best to overt representations of sexuality. It is interesting that repetition doesn't seem to extinguish or diminish the value of favourite fantasies in men. It might be thought that living out the same scene time and again might become boring, especially as it's based on visual components of sexual relationships, as opposed to romantic and emotional ones, but this hasn't been found to be the case. Females have their favourites, too, but they tend to be more emotionally complex in content compared with the more anatomically and visually explicit material enjoyed by men.

RECOUNTING YOUR FANTASIES

Many couples find that knowing about each other's fantasies can help a relationship. Such knowledge dispels fear: the fear that makes you feel odd or likely to be rejected. Although airing a fantasy can have negative side-effects (*see* pages 153-155), if told cautiously it need not. Partners who are aware of their own fantasies and their significance can use their knowledge to enhance their sex life and their relationship.

In Part Two I describe how such themes arise in the psyche and what can be learned about yourself, your partners and your relationships from such insights. It's important to treat this new-found knowledge with respect. It can be fun to explore your thoughts, but be careful not to dump theories on to your partner, who may not feel easy with them. Rather, try to offer a thought to chew on, perhaps alongside evidence from your personal knowledge.

By opening up to fantasy in this way, you should be able to explore many areas within your relationship that have nothing to do with sex. Talk about what this means to you both. See how the new knowledge can help enrich your love life, perhaps by acting out a fantasy or something close to it. Think about your role as parents, if you have children, and see how your new understanding can help you be more effective. There's much to be learned from exploring how fantasies can colour behaviour at work, at play and in all areas of life. Try not to overdo the 'therapy' between you; balance your own interpretations of your partner's fantasies with a healthy willingness to open yourself up to scrutiny, too.

The other main function of Part Two is to illustrate what other people fantasize about. When I explore different fantasy themes with my patients they almost always say how surprising it is that there are so many themes which don't interest them one bit. This is to be expected, given the highly personalized nature of fantasies. But this gives rise to a dilemma for me as a therapist, which might become clear when reading the next chapter.

The subjects of some of their fantasies – most commonly those about animals or children – upset many people. It makes sense, if my clinical experience is anything to go by, to tread lightly in such areas, because I find the fantasies that arouse most hostility or anger frequently turn out to be the ones that the individual's unconscious most needs. A good example of this was a patient who read a fantasy book called *The Story of O* by Pauline Reage (Corgi 1972), which contained considerable sado-masochistic activity, including anal sex. She was so furious with me for suggesting she read it that she threw it out of the window one day in disgust.

I was understandably keen to explore her response to this best seller and felt intuitively that change was just around the corner. In fact, it took her only a few weeks consciously to acknowledge that such matters were in fact so arousing that she couldn't cope with the degree of sexual excitement they produced. Her fears of being taken over by her arousal, or that she might become some sort of sex maniac, were so great in her unconscious that she rejected this powerful source of fantasy-induced pleasure out of hand.

These paradoxes are much harder to handle in the home than in the consulting room, but they're present in both and have to be addressed. By saying this I'm not suggesting that the woman who reads a fantasy about sex with an animal and feels sick should be encouraged to make it a regular favourite. This would be foolish. However, it's sensible for people to monitor their partners' bodily response to such apparently disturbing fantasy themes and believe these responses, rather than what their partners say they feel. The unconscious never lies to the genitals. The erect penis or the wet vagina reveal much more than any eloquent speech.

If you've never had a conscious fantasy, Part Two should be a great help. I find in practice that many people, women especially, who say they don't fantasize, start to do so, and readily, once they have some models to go by. Quite a few people ask me what they should fantasize about. It's impossible to say because I'm not, at that stage, deeply enough involved with their unconscious, and even if I were, I wouldn't presume to suggest a theme. But by reading the fantasies of others, such individuals soon get the hang of fantasizing and start to embroider their own stories based, perhaps, on ones they've read.

This can also be helpful if you're heavily involved in a fantasy that doesn't feel right, for some reason. Knowing what to substitute for it can be tricky if you've little access to erotic literature or videos. This collection may help to solve the problem.

Please try to be compassionate and tolerant when you read Part Two. There will be subjects that disgust and amaze you, but please bear in mind that the fantasist who creates them is not you. If your unique sexual past and present match sufficiently with those of any of the fantasists, you will probably find their stories adequately arousing to build into your own fantasy life. If they don't, you will probably never have anything in common with the teller. This doesn't make you strange or inhibited, just different.

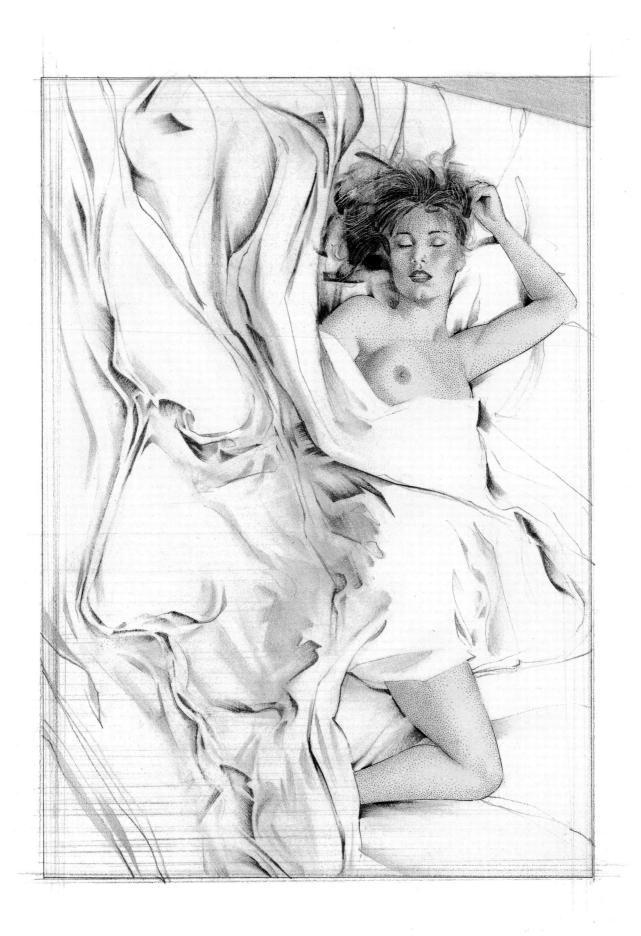

PART TWO

Understanding Your Fantasies

All human fantasies and day-dreams originate in the unconscious. You may become aware of them when your unconscious 'censor' allows some through when you sleep, or when something happens to bring them to the surface in your waking life. No two people's fantasies are identical, although there are common themes. In this part of the book I look at more than 40 of the most important and popular of these, describe their erotic elements and interpret them to reveal what a fantasy tells its creator about his or her sex life. My aim is to make you feel at ease with your own and your partner's fantasies, and with the idea of fantasizing. Better understanding has the effect of enriching both loving and sexual relationships.

INTRODUCTION

The fantasy themes covered in this part of the book are common – in various different guises – to both men and women. When I use a male as the protagonist I don't mean to imply that a woman can't enjoy such a fantasy, or vice versa. It may simply be that the type of fantasy I describe is very much more popular with men than with women.

Readers may wonder how I came by the fantasies I report in this part of the book. Two are reproduced as they were written to me, and have been used with permission. The vast majority, however, are composite fantasies embodying a number of common sub-themes in any given area. There is space in this book to describe only one fantasy per subject, and a single real-life fantasy would usually not have incorporated the many and complex themes that run as undercurrents in almost every fantasy type. Using composite fantasies also protects many patients from having their very private lives paraded in minute detail.

I arrived at most of the fantasies by one or more of several methods. First, some people tell me their fantasies directly as a story, face to face, when talking about other matters to do with sex and relationships. Most, though, find this quite difficult to do in any detail, so I use one or more of several other techniques. The most fruitful of these is a sort of hypnotic regression method. In this, and in fantasy-training sessions, I find that people are much more ready to share what they really use as fantasy material. Their internal censor is off duty and true fantasy material surfaces readily. I can also make suggestions, or question certain unlikely-sounding parts of a fantasy, and by doing so arrive at what is really going on.

Another method is to ask an individual to write a two-page script for an X-rated video. Often what transpires is the individual's pure fantasy, straight from the unconscious, unfiltered and unexamined. This provides us with valuable work for several therapy sessions and can be a real eye-opener for the person's partner, too.

Of course, I have also used fantasies of my own and those of people I have known well, if they illustrate a point.

People are always asking me whether what I hear are 'real' fantasies, or whether they are somehow created specially for my ears. I suspect some of the fantasies reported in self-selected responses to researchers' magazine and newspaper requests for fantasy material; the one-to-one, trusting relationship developed in a meaningful therapeutic alliance is much more likely to produce true fantasies than embellished stories, even though they are really fantasy *tales*. What I'm interested in is not simply what people *can* conjure up in their imagination, but what really *affects* them. This means that the material has to come largely from the unconscious. On occasions, sleeping dreams reveal the basis of an individual's erotic fantasy life better than anything else.

Also, bear in mind when reading this part of the book that most people use parts of their favourite fantasies, as well as the whole story, and that many people vary the story slightly from episode to episode to keep the interest up and prevent boredom. I often find this when referring back to something someone told me a few weeks ago. He or she will say, 'Oh, I've gone on from there; I now fantasize about . . .'. Or, having shared with me an early fantasy and obtained 'permission' to make it their own, they go on to explore further, but keep their new story from me, and possibly their partner, so as to increase its private value to them.

The language used by some of my characters might shock some readers. But when people recount their fantasies, especially in writing, they use much more raunchy words and phrases than they usually do, except, perhaps, in the throes of love-making. I never try to sanitize my patients' language and I find that for them to be at ease I have to adopt the style of speech they prefer.

The term 'sexual intercourse' in such fantasy settings as I describe simply doesn't have the same ring as the word 'fucking'. Few of my patients would use the word 'vulva' or 'penis'; many feel more comfortable with the slang terms, 'cunt' and 'prick'. I hope that this vernacular approach in recounting people's fantasies doesn't offend you.

In most of the fantasy themes I describe in this part of the book, I begin by discussing and analyzing the main ideas behind each theme, and go on to reproduce an example of a typical fantasy to illustrate these ideas. Having said this, the first three topics are so wide-reaching there can be no typical fantasy to reproduce. Clearly, 'sex with a current partner' could mean anything.

While I have deliberately tried to exclude fantasies that describe dangerous practices that could harm anyone, it is probably sensible for me to point out that these are *fantasies*. If you find yourself aroused by them and want to act them out with your partner, please be very cautious.

SEX WITH A CURRENT PARTNER

The fact that the commonest reported fantasy themes involve an individual's current sexual partner might at first seem unlikely. After all, aren't fantasies supposed to be about the unattainable, the dream partner? Of course they can be and are, but neither of these ideas need rule out day-dreams or fantasies about an available flesh-and-blood lover. If you have something good, it makes sense to use it to enhance your arousal.

On the other hand, few people can honestly say that their partner is exactly what they want, in every dimension of the relationship. An individual who is great in bed might be less loving and considerate in everyday life than his or her partner would like. The partner might then fantasize about loving and considerate behaviour to make up for the deficit.

When it comes to sexual and romantic pursuits individuals will go only so far – there is always something they cannot bring themselves to do. Sometimes, their final position falls short of what their partner wants or needs. Fantasy is a device that can be used to make up for this shortfall.

Every one-to-one relationship has its past; specific occasions stick in the mind to be recalled and cherished later. Fantasy is a wonderful way of celebrating these precious times. A well of romantic and sexual memories is available to sustain a relationship suffering from drought – I see the popularity of current-partner fantasies as a way of shoring up a relationship and of being reassured of its worth. Fantasizing about someone who is physically or emotionally absent for some reason can carry a partner through until his or her return.

Fantasizing about one another also helps bond lovers together in a troubled world that often seems to be the enemy of the one-to-one relationship. The pleasures and intimacies shared; the secret society of two; the knowledge that your partner understands you better than anyone else; the level of trust; the absence of guilt; the anxiety-free play; these and much more make fantasizing about a current partner safe, exciting and valuable.

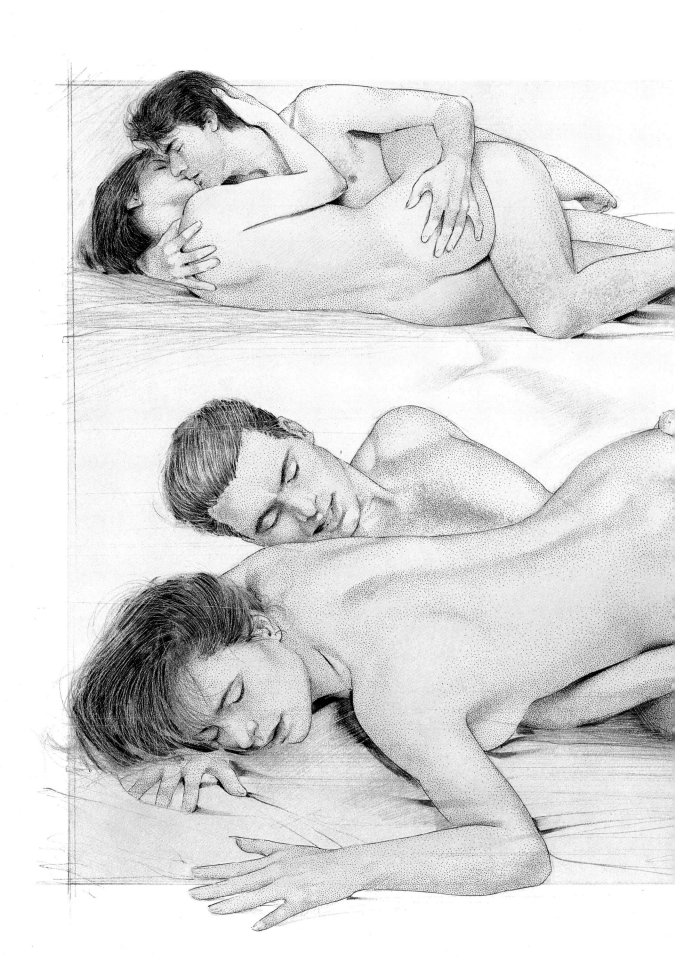

And in a growing relationship there is room for development within the safe confines of this partnership. Advances in sexual activity can first be rehearsed in fantasy, before being made a reality. Adversity and sexual failure can also be accommodated by recalling better times, perhaps even out loud, with a partner.

Many a flaccid penis is saved by a man's partner, or, indeed, by its owner, recalling an especially successful and enjoyable encounter.

Contrary, therefore, to what many readers may think, it is possible – and, arguably, even desirable – to have a fantasy life that is kept largely within the boundaries of a one-to-one relationship. This dispels any concerns about 'adultery in the mind'. It is, and will probably remain, the most popular fantasy theme.

SEX WITH A PREVIOUS PARTNER

'Memories are made of this', as the old song goes. Most people like to relive the good times past, not just when things are going badly in the present, but in fond memory of the past for its own sake. There is nothing wrong with this. All individuals are products of their pasts and it is impossible to get away from the fact.

Our sexual past will not go away. It is an integral part of who we are. Making love while fantasizing about a past lover revives these powerful memories and enriches arousal.

Some people, feeling a little adulterous in such fantasies, are guilty about them. Ways of overcoming guilt are described on page 151. Suffice it to say here that for many people there will always be pleasantly memorable episodes that can provide a rich store of themes on which to draw to enrich their current fantasy life.

Research shows that people don't tend to marry the lover they were most passionately involved with in their search for a permanent partner. They play safe, settling for what they consider the most suitable attributes. This can mean that some people find memories of past lovers a more potent sexual turn-on than thoughts of their current one.

When I discuss this with couples, one or other sometimes becomes quiet and acts hurt, or worse. But the fact is that people choose a partner for many complex and usually unconscious reasons. One of these has to do with their partner's past, and this includes his or her past partners. It is irrational to say 'I love you as you are', yet somehow edit out the bits of a partner's past that are hard to accept. The past has made the partner what he or she is today; the person we like and love.

However, there are dangers. Lingering in the past or dwelling mainly on old flames rather than your current lover can be detrimental to a relationship, so it makes sense to seek professional help to sort things out. Many people know intuitively when this is happening to their partner. Some people have even told me outright that they know their partner is fantasizing about a previous lover, perhaps soon after an affair is ended, while making love to them. How couples handle this is up to them, but there is a good case to be made for bringing it all out in the open and getting it out of the fantasist's system. Fantasy thrives on secrecy. Uncovering it in this way can knock such a fantasy on the head faster than any other way I know.

With the wisdom of hindsight, many people tend to embroider sexual events from the past in fantasies, just as they embellish their non-sexual memories. 'The good old days' are well known to have been far better than the present, even if, in truth, they were not. But it is wise to remember that distance lends enchantment to the view if you find yourself becoming obsessed in your fantasies with an old flame. Such nostalgia is valuable in moderation, but it can get out of control if you're unrealistic. I find it interesting and useful when this becomes a problem for people to help them remember that previous partners are 'previous' for a good reason, or perhaps for many reasons. Had they been as marvellous as they appear in fantasies, perhaps they wouldn't be past partners.

Lastly, some people relive old relationships in their fantasies to complete what they see as unfinished business. In this sense, fantasies of this kind are healing, completing and helpful.

NEW SEX POSITIONS

This type of fantasy is perhaps more commonly found in men than women, but it always comes near the top when either sex is asked to recount favourite fantasies.

Sex in long-term partnerships can become rather samey after a while, no matter how good the relationship. Sexual boredom is, it seems, the plague of modern long-term relationships, but this is hardly surprising, given the length of marriages today compared with only a century ago. Today's couples who stay together can expect to do so for about 52 years if people continue to marry in their mid-twenties and die in their late seventies.

But the desire for novelty is based on more than just the longevity of lasting partnerships. People today live in a changing world, where novelty is revered. It's ironic, therefore, that most happy couples make love in the same two or three positions for almost the whole of their sexual lives together. Yet there is still a thrill to be derived from trying out new love-making positions. The delight of discovery that most people enjoyed in their teens and early twenties can be relived through experimentation with new positions in fact or in fantasy. People tell me that on occasions experiencing this can be like having a completely new lover.

It's also worth noting that fantasies about sex in unfamiliar positions are sometimes created consciously or unconsciously because they enable an individual to be unfaithful with a long-term partner by acting out a new scenario as if he or she were someone else. This topic is discussed in page 68.

So by and large, whether in fact or fantasy,

experimentation with new positions for sex can be useful and growth-enhancing. Unfortunately this is not always so. Some men, particularly in mid-life, become sexually tiresome as they seek to try out all kinds of new positions. To some extent this has much to do with what they fear they have lost, never had, or are missing out on. But, conversely, such activity can result from much more devious workings of the mind, as some men use it – usually quite unconsciously – to test their partner's love for them.

Many a man has told me that if his wife or girlfriend really loved him she would be, or do, some special thing. In a culture that links sex so closely with love, many women say they will have sex only with a man they love. Such men can therefore be forgiven for believing that the sign of being really loved by a woman is that she will do exactly what they want sexually.

Despite appearances to the contrary, modern sexuality has a distinctly unadventurous tinge, so it should come as no surprise to find that many men test their relationship and their women's love for them by making demands for new sexual positions. Is she like the liberated women he reads about? If not, why not?

Some people of either sex make demands for new sex positions unconsciously to rock the marital boat, to create an issue which can then be used as evidence to support the argument that they are not suited. Their incompatibility really occurs principally in other areas of their lives, but it has become fashionable to point to failures in the bedroom as irrefutable evidence that 'we can't get on'.

As with many aspects of sex, this one is a matter of balance, both in the conscious and the unconscious. Individuals need novelty or they become bored, yet to have too much becomes a nuisance because they can't tell where they stand in the relationship. This balance between the familiar, safe and known, and the novel, anxiety-inducing and unknown, is one that many successful couples sort out for themselves, often unwittingly. But the lives of millions of others are plagued by the problem asserting itself in hidden ways.

There will always be sex positions with which some individuals cannot cope. For example, a woman who has a hang-up about her fat bottom may be unable to tolerate rear-entry positions. A man with problems keeping an erection may find that woman-on-top arrangements make him fail sexually. In fantasy, such positions can be explored safely, even, perhaps, with a current partner. As with all other fantasies, this can be a good rehearsal ground before attempting something one day when you feel especially loving or uninhibited.

For a few couples, certain sex positions are impossible for various reasons – if one partner is physically handicapped in some way, for example, perhaps with arthritic hips. A man with angina may be unable to take much of a dominant role if he's worried about his heart, yet he can quite happily fantasize about positions he would like to adopt but can't for health reasons.

Other factors, not just physical health, can stand in the way of certain sexual positions and relegate them to the realm of fantasy. Emotional and relationship factors control things, too. Most women say they feel safest and most feminine in the classic missionary position, which, they also claim, is the most romantic. On the other hand, some women would like to get on top of their man from time to time, but can't because it intimidates him. For some of their partners this position is their least favourite, because although they may need the woman to be active and in control, many men are not able to accept this need when it comes to it. They would benefit from realizing that they need the woman, if only from time to time, to control things, and to adopt new positions that facilitate her taking control. If dealing with these issues in real life is difficult, threatening, or even impossible because the woman won't comply or the man can't bring himself to ask for what he wants, fantasy can come to the rescue.

ROMANTIC SEX

M any women enjoy fantasies of romantic sex. It is their most popular fantasy type or, more accurately, the most readily admitted to on questionnaires. Men have romantic fantasies, too, but not nearly so often; so, for simplicity, I shall confine myself to discussing this subject in the context of females.

Right from the earliest days of a girl's life within her family, romantic sex is stressed and valued, often at the expense of other types of sex. Sex is closely associated with romance in a girl's mind from well before she starts dating.

Fiction for girls and, of course, romantic fiction for women, emphasizes all this, enhances it further, and encourages the link between romantic notions and sexual needs and their expression.

This subject is vast and fascinating but I can deal with it only very superficially in this book. Romantic fiction is a thriving area of publishing in the Western world. There are at least 20 million loyal readers in the USA and the popularity of romantic fiction has spread to almost every Western country.

The central core of such fiction is that the heroine is physically attractive, emotionally open and sensual. The whole story is told through her eyes. These qualities are both her problem and her salvation because not only do they 'get her into trouble' with men but they also give her the power to manipulate the hero and other powerful men around her.

Plotlines change as society moves on. Large romantic fiction publishers are now returning to rather less permissive storylines since the AIDS scare. Bodices are now being ripped rather less readily. Yet, overall, the heroines of such stories end up with their men after a struggle for emotional dominance. The action takes place in a sort of 'pornotopia', an exotic locale that helps the reader escape from her humdrum life and makes the events even more acceptable and exciting.

Much had been written about the triviality of such novels. They are, it is claimed, simply a way for women to get what they so passionately desire but cannot have in daily life – a romantic man. My view is somewhat less condemnatory than this. I see romantic fiction as soft porn for women. Just as men lust after sexy women in the pages of girlie magazines, so some women lust after romantic men in their fiction. Both types of material are equally 'fantastic', in the purist sense of the word.

That this is not simply a fanciful notion can be demonstrated by looking at studies of the sexual arousal of women reading such novels. Even though they claim not to be aroused, in fact they are, and sometimes greatly so, as their genital responses prove when measured in laboratory experiments.

Studies of women who read romantic fiction find that they are just like other women. The only key feature seems to be age: more younger women read romance than do older women. On balance, readers have been found to be more preoccupied with sexual behaviour than non-readers. Many people imagine that women use these books as an alternative to real-life sex, but this is probably not true. Older readers of the genre have twice as much sex as non-readers, according to one study, which also found that readers who are housewives are more satisfied with their sex lives than non-readers. Many women who enjoy these books use their reading to enhance their fantasies during sexual intercourse, while non-readers seldom or never do so.

It used to be said that women do not respond to frankly erotic material, only to romantic stories. This has long since been disproved. Women react in exactly the same way as men to erotic tapes or videos. Such 'full-frontal' sexuality is still hard for many women to accept, at least at a conscious level, because it's too obvious and confronts their lifelong notion that to be sexually acceptable they should be passive and romantic.

Although women's roles and attitudes are changing in society, things are not moving all that quickly in the unconscious. The old restrictive notions of the past still hold sway and many millions of women are not yet sufficiently comfortable with their sexuality to be able to relate to it directly. They require the romantic metaphor to sanitize it and reduce the anxiety that would otherwise result.

But confusion reigns as the traditional romantic fictional male hero, strong, silent, unemotional and domineering, takes his place among the New Men of the nineties. How all this will come to rest in fact and fantasy only time will tell.

Romantic fantasies take many forms, but very often they include an exotic location – sometimes one the owner has visited. Eleanor's fantasy shows that even though it is highly romantic it doesn't have to be devoid of a genital component – or even of love-making. There is never any copulation or fucking in romantic fantasies. It is always beautiful love-making: true intercourse, in the sense of an intimate, soul-to-soul sexual connection with a loved an cherished partner.

HEAVEN IN HIS ARMS

I'm on vacation in Florida with a girlfriend, and we meet these two guys. One obviously likes me and makes a pass at me almost as soon as we meet. Over the next few days we get to talk a lot and we seem to have masses in common. The fantasy starts one night after a lovely meal outside at a beachside restaurant. We've both had just enough to drink to make us relaxed, yet not enough to spoil things. He's exceptionally tender, looks longingly at me and keeps taking my hand.

When we've finished eating he suggests that we go for a midnight walk along the beach away from the restaurant and the people. It's idyllic. The air is warm and ripples through the thin material of my cotton dress. I'm wearing only the tiniest of briefs underneath and feel so deliciously sensuous. We walk arm in arm, stopping now and again to kiss. He holds my head gently in his large, tanned hands and kisses me all over my neck, ears and face. I feel myself melting with a warm glow that seeps through the whole of my body from top to bottom.

As he kisses me I run my hands over his hard, muscular back and sense a certain kind of helplessness as I know I'm going to get carried away into romantic oblivion before long. I know it's hopeless to fight it and really don't want to.

We walk a little further before he stops and turns to me and, looking directly into my eyes, starts to take off my dress. I'm a bit shy but it's nearly dark, the only light coming from the moon, which isn't very full. As I allow my dress to fall around my ankles he murmurs his admiration at the sight of my firm, brown body ... most of which he has seen before anyway in my bikini. Somehow it feels so different, though, tonight.

Before I know what's happening he starts to cover my body with kisses and caresses, so that I feel I'm being overwhelmed by waves of delicious feelings. I slowly take his shirt off and start to kiss and lick his chest. He tastes so good, so male. His smell and his strength make me want him.

But he's not rushing me. He takes off his slacks and sandals and now, perfectly naked, takes me to the water's edge and leads me in. At first the shock of the cold startles me a little, but soon it's up to my waist and he reaches down to remove my panties. We are now totally naked in the warm water. Several hundred yards away people are eating their meals at the restaurant and I can't help wondering what they'd think if they knew what we were up to. Being so private, so intimate, yet not that far away from other people, is a real turn on.

With one firm move he brings my waist against his and then slowly and lovingly leans me backward until I'm lying flat on the water. He opens my legs, which takes little effort as I'm aching to put them round his waist. Within seconds he is in me, slowly at first, then forcefully as he penetrates more deeply.

The sensations of the water and him inside me are almost too much to bear. I cry out a little with pleasure.

'Are you all right?' he asks. 'I'm in heaven,' I reply, as he finds his natural rhythm and holds me strongly, my body supported by the surface of the water.

After what seems like hours of pleasure I climax as I have never done before. He holds me tight and then, lifting me bodily out of the water as if I were a doll, takes me back to the sand, lays me down and hugs me to him, holding me in his strong, muscular arms as I drift off to sleep.

NON-GENITAL LOVE-MAKING

Fantasies of this kind are commonly found in both sexes. They can be a pleasant change from frankly genital reveries; and they may be used by certain people as alternatives because their unconscious will not allow them to deal head-on with matters concerned with the genitals.

Young men with little experience of real-life sex often have such fantasies as they explore their new-found sexual 'toys'. A touch of a girl's breast, a kiss, a glimpse of her panties and other non-genital activities can provide fantasy material for months, or even years. The inhibited of any age find that non-genital fantasies keep them safe, yet provide arousal.

Common themes include touching and being touched; caressing a woman's breasts; massaging one another; cuddling and kissing; and other pleasures. With recent scares about too headlong a rush into genital activity, the awareness of herpes and AIDS, and the linking of cervical cancer in young women with the number of their sexual partners, I suspect that more people are using non-genital sex in reality and in fantasy than they did ten years ago.

Tony's fantasy is fairly typical of its kind. He uses it because it suits his current relationship:

THE PLEASURE OF TOUCHING

I'm in my early twenties and haven't had much sexual experience to speak of. My favourite fantasy is about cuddling my girl and then massaging her all over for a long time. We're in front of the fire at her place. Her parents are out for the evening. We explore one another's bodies and I massage her.

In real life she doesn't want to have sex before we marry and in my fantasy I try to pleasure her in every way I can, short of entering her. I start with her back, go on to her stomach and legs, and then massage her breasts and nipples. By now she's usually hot and ready to have an orgasm, so I play with her breasts some more and run my fingers all over her body to tease her.

Even though I don't touch her genitals at all, she climaxes and is thankful that I don't make her go further than she wants. In fact, this suits me quite well too, because I'm rather shy about my penis and I'd rather not disappoint her. Just massaging her like this in my fantasy means I can please her without having to do anything else.

ORAL SEX

Always very near the top of the list with men, this is an increasingly common fantasy favourite with women, too. In an age when women are making more demands on their men for sexual results, it is provable that the tongue is mightier than the penis when it comes to inducing orgasms from stimulation of the clitoris.

Cunnilingus is not just a way of taking the pressure off the penis: it confers considerable power on the man as he gives his partner predictable, shuddering orgasms. For the man who married a 'nice' girl, oral sex enables him to transform a virginal wife into the abandoned whore he always wanted. 'Going down' on a woman is now so commonplace that females complain to me if their man will not do it. Thirty years ago they complained when he did.

Everyone has the potential to give and receive oral pleasure, right from the earliest days as infants at the breast or bottle. Exploring with the mouth continues past infancy in many pastimes: the pleasures of food, smoking and drinking are obvious manifestations of this in adult life.

Making love using the mouth is very obvious when kissing, sucking, nibbling and licking a partner, and fantasy life, like real life, is peppered with oro-genital contact. From a man's point of view it's an extremely intimate and loving thing for a woman to be involved in. Whether she fellates him (men's favourite) or allows him to caress her genitals orally, he feels truly loved and valued as a male. The vulnerability of either sex in such situations obviously calls for considerable trust, and it can be this reassurance that the fantasist really seeks. Reliving this love and trust in fantasy can enhance and reinforce the value of a sexual partner.

In fantasy, oral sex can be made perfect in a way that cannot happen, perhaps, in real life. Many women, for example, do not like to swallow semen, even if they will kiss and suck their man's penis. As a result many men's fantasies of oral sex involve a woman, perhaps their partner, swallowing their semen with delight and uninhibited pleasure. Similarly, some men will not go down on their woman and they, in their turn, can make up for this in their fantasy life.

Phil's fantasy started some years ago after picking up a woman for sex when he was away on business:

ELECTRICAL TURN-ON

In my fantasy I'm staying in a hotel on business when I see a fantastic woman at the bar. I know I'm on to a good thing because she was there the night before and is obviously alone, like me.

I start to chat her up and she lets drop that she'd like someone to mend the plug on the hair-drier in her room. I offer to do it. She asks me to wait down at the bar while she goes to phone someone from her room and to come to see her in ten minutes' time. The next ten minutes drag by as I start to anticipate what might happen. I look at my watch about 20 times, order another drink for courage, and go to the elevators. The tenth floor seems a mile away, with the whole world getting on and off at each floor.

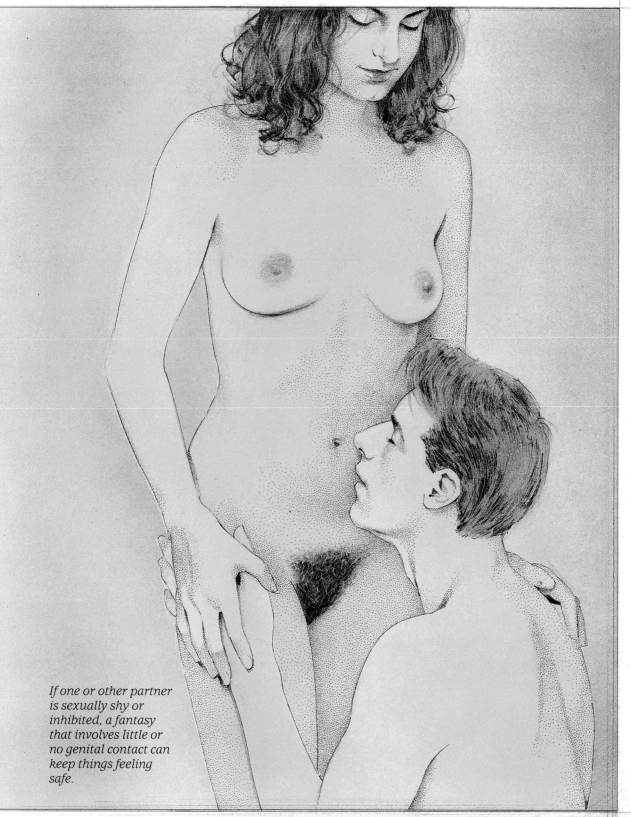

If one or other partner is sexually shy or inhibited, a fantasy that involves little or no genital contact can keep things feeling safe.

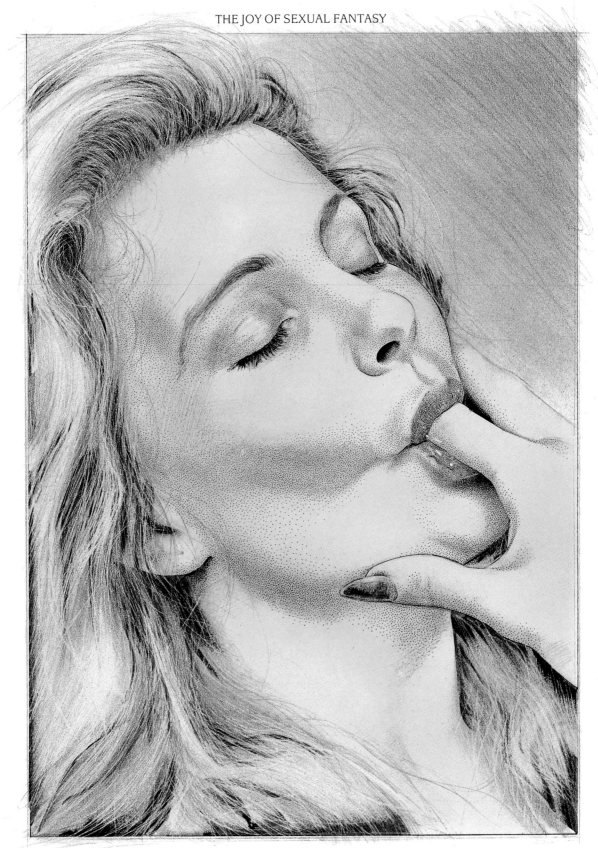

I get out of the elevator and find her room. I knock gingerly on the door, somewhat apprehensive.

She opens the door. Imagine my surprise to see her standing there dressed only in her negligée. She looks fantastic. She motions for me to come in.

'Thanks. Where's the drier?' I ask.

'I'll get it for you,' she says. She goes to the dressing table and hands it to me.

I play with it for a few seconds. 'I can't *see* anything wrong with it,' I say, not having a clue; 'but there might be a loose connection in the plug. Have you got a nail file?'

'Here,' she replies, giving it to me. 'While you fix it I'll just take a shower.'

So there's me fiddling away with the nail file, undoing the plug, while she showers within feet of me, this gorgeous female I've never met before. In fact, the wire *is* loose and it's easily mended. She comes out of the shower clad only in a large bath towel, drying herself and looking so sexy that I could have jumped on her there and then.

'I've fixed it.' I say proudly.

'Thought you would,' she smiles; 'now let's see if it works.' Without a blink she throws the towel off on to the floor and lays down stark naked on the bed.

'Perhaps you'd like to try it out here,' she says, pointing to her pubic hair.

I don't need asking twice. I'm on the bed playing the current of warm air over her fanny and gently running my fingers through her hair before she's finished asking. The warm air soon begins to have its desired effect and she starts to breathe heavily. Her legs open slightly, and she begins to caress her breasts.

'It's too hot,' she moans after a while. 'Cool me down now.'

I take my cue from her and, getting down between her legs, I go down on her fresh pussy and cool her hot, aching clitoris with my wet tongue.

'How's that?' I ask, raising my head for a moment. But she's in another world.

Within seconds I'm nuzzling her sweet-smelling cunt again and caressing her little knob to a climax. Her body writhes as she clasps her thighs so hard around my head I think she'll screw it off. But it's such bliss that I keep on tonguing her more and more as she writhes and tosses from side to side, trying to push my tongue deeper into her vagina. The wetness of my spit and her juices mingle as we roll together, moaning and wallowing in one another.

By this stage of the fantasy I've usually come. In fact, if I'm really aroused I can sometimes ejaculate by the time I start to use the hair-drier, so powerful is the fantasy.

The pleasure she is obtaining from her mouth is plain to see. Whether her fantasy involves sucking or kissing a penis hardly matters . . . it is the oral joy she seeks.

BEING IRRESISTIBLE

This common female fantasy is also sometimes enjoyed by males. Most people like to think they are desirable. If you are sexually attractive enough to be overwhelmed by someone simply because you're so irresistible, it's easy to deny responsibility for what follows. This sort of fantasy has always been popular with women because in Western culture it has been unacceptable for a woman to be a party to her own seduction. In more recent times this has started to change; now women often take the sexual initiative, both in and out of bed.

Nevertheless, the cultural norm is that a woman who initiates sexual activities with a man – especially one who isn't her partner – is a floozy or a whore, so women wishing to do so have had to find ways that are congruent with these unconscious beliefs. Clearly, being so irresistible that a man can't keep his hands off you is one effective way of achieving this. 'After all,' such women say to me, 'I can't help being so attractive, sexy, adorable (or whatever), it's just how I am.'

Both sexes can be inhibited in a way that stops them from seeking or actualizing their conscious or unconscious sexual drives. For such an individual, fantasies of being 'taken over' are very exciting. The responsibility for the 'dirty deed' rests firmly with the perpetrator and the fantasist can relax, enjoy the sex and do so from the safe standpoint of a pawn in the sexual game. Someone else is conducting the orchestra – all the individual has to do is comply.

Sometimes such a fantasy originates from the underlying, usually unconscious, fear that the owner is in fact highly resistible. I see this in people of both sexes who have poor self-esteem or who are socially inept. Sometimes a young, inexperienced man who, in real life, can't attract women will become irresistible in his fantasies. While this serves him well during an episode of masturbation, looked at in the long term it probably doesn't do him any favours, because it confirms his imaginary view that with little or no effort women will flock to him for sex. Alas, many such men tell me, their real world is nothing like this.

Peter shows how such a fantasy can be used to obtain what an individual wants, but in reality can't have:

An Urgent Meeting

In real life I'm a middle manager in a major manufacturing company. I have to deal a lot with a fantastic-looking woman who looks after our PR account. My work involves going to the agency to see her and her team, so we meet almost every week for one reason or another. In real life she's married and is totally unavailable, but in my fantasy things are rather different.

My favourite day-dream about her is that one day I go to the agency and see her going up the stairs as I enter the hallway of the building. She's looking immensely desirable. Her auburn hair cascades in gentle waves to come to rest on her shoulders. She's dressed in a black business suit that shows off her curves seductively, and her white blouse is slightly see-through, so I can tell she isn't wearing a bra: there's just a hint of nipple visible through the fabric.

She stands on the stairs as if to mount them, her right foot on a higher stair than her left, caught in mid-step as she stops to greet me, her legs slightly apart.

'Hello, Peter,' she smiles warmly, 'you're early for the meeting.'

'I know,' I say. 'I wanted to talk to you about something before the others arrive.' My eyes are fixed on her legs. Her short skirt is riding up to well above the middle of her thighs. She leans down over the bannister to talk to me. I can see down the front of her blouse to confirm that she is bra-less.

'Why don't you come up and we can talk?' she motions, straightening up.

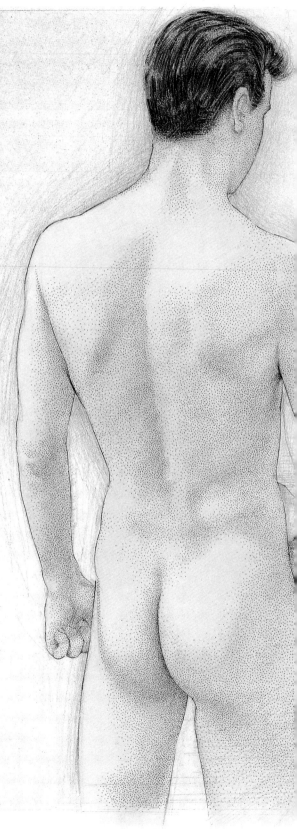

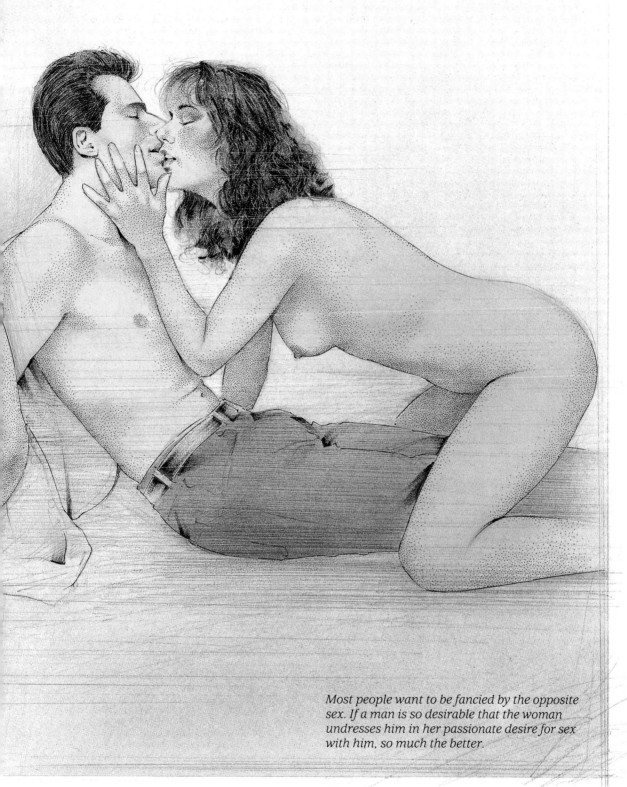

Most people want to be fancied by the opposite sex. If a man is so desirable that the woman undresses him in her passionate desire for sex with him, so much the better.

'Thanks,' I gasp, realizing that she had bent down quite deliberately so I could see her tits.

I follow her up the stairs, acutely aware of her behind encased in the beautifully tailored cloth of her skirt. She wriggles more than is necessary, or at least I imagine she does.

'You go into the conference room and I'll be with you in a sec,' she says as she disappears into her office.

I make myself at home at the large, glass-topped table and lay out my papers. Very soon she is back with two coffees, a pile of papers and a broad grin.

'We never seem to have any time together,' she purrs, looking directly into my eyes in a way that completely throws me. 'And that's a shame because you're really quite a guy and I'd like to get to know you better.'

I splutter into my coffee, trying to hide my amazement. 'But,' I blurt out, 'I thought you were spoken for. What about your husband?'

'He's a rotten bastard,' she snaps. 'Always off with some tart or other. I'd leave him if it weren't for the damned good lifestyle he gives me. Now you know how to treat a lady.'

She is now sitting down at the opposite side of the table, arranging her papers and sipping her coffee. As she hands me a paper she brushes her hand against mine and holds the document just that split second too long, the cue that tells me she's making a pass at me.

We talk shop for a while and as we do so I can't help noticing that her skirt is riding right up her thighs. She edges her bottom to the front of the chair to reveal her thighs and, to my astonished delight, the fact that she's wearing no panties.

She sits there calmly talking business and slowly parting her thighs to reveal her crotch, all clearly visible through the glass table top. I can hardly believe my eyes. This vision of loveliness that I thought was totally unavailable is throwing herself at me in a quite outrageous way.

She begins to notice the effect she's having and goes to the door and locks it. Coming over to me she beckons for me to stand up. Slowly she unzips my fly and takes out my prick. Deftly, and with great, almost professional, skill, she kneels down and sucks it expertly until I come in her mouth.

At that moment someone passes the door. She straightens up, I hastily make myself decent and she unlocks the door to let in the other members of the meeting.

MAKING LOVE IN NEW PLACES

Various studies have looked at this subject, and interviewees often claim that they would very much like to have sex in their living room, bathroom, kitchen or garden, as a change from the bedroom. Although some people have fantasies of exotic locations (this is especially true of women's romantic fantasies), most of those who indulge in this kind of reverie think about places far nearer home. Boredom and the yearning for novelty and change are at the heart of this fantasy.

Making love in a new location can add spice to a relationship that is flagging in fact or fantasy. For some people, a change of place in which to have sex is almost as exciting as a change of partner.

Love-making out of doors – in semi-public places, in tents and so on – has the added excitement that being naughty in public has for a child. The thrill of the new and the fear of discovery add to the arousal.

Dot's fantasy is an extension of her real life, using a man she meets in her work as a barmaid in a pub in South London, and creating an exciting scene which contrasts starkly with her real-life, boring husband:

PLAYTIME IN THE GARDEN

In real life I'm a barmaid working in our local. It's great fun, but most of all it gets me out of the house away from the old man and the kids and makes a few pounds for the family.

The bit I like best, though, is meeting the guys. Otherwise, quite honestly, I think I'd go stark raving mad at the thought of being married to my old man for the next 40 years.

Anyway, there's this great guy who comes in most nights and I know he lusts after me something rotten. Of course the best bit is that I go for him in a big way myself.

My fantasy starts with him coming in to drink one night and then staying right to the

Sex and water have very ancient connections in the collective unconscious. Any location or setting in which water can be used erotically can be a fantasy winner.

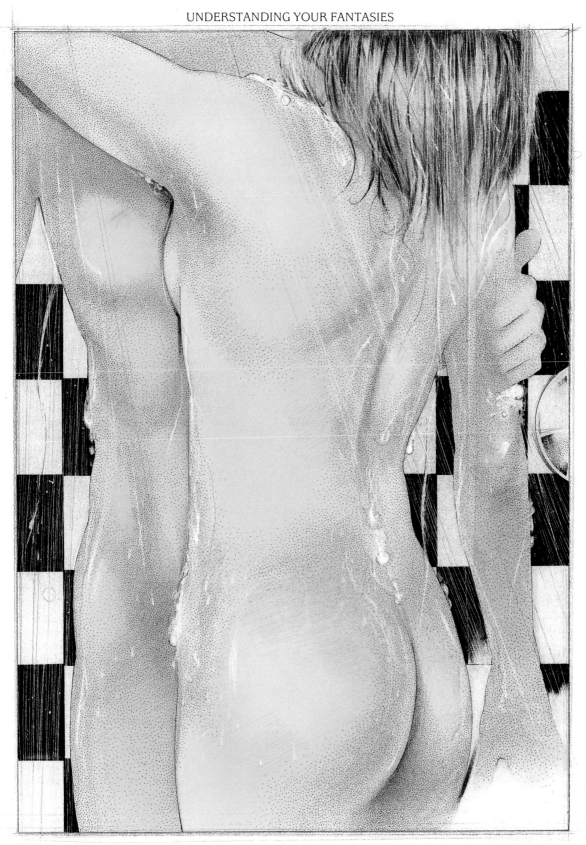

end. He hangs around, which is unusual for him. As I clear up when everyone else has gone, he starts to chat me up in a very obvious sexy way. He knows I'm married, but also knows that I'm open to offers if they're good.

'Fancy coming outside for a walk to cool off, Dot?' he asks.

'OK,' I say. 'Let me just finish these glasses and cash up and I'll be with you.'

My jobs done, I follow him out into the pub garden. It's dark and completely deserted. All the customers have gone and the landlord and his wife, who live in, have gone out visiting.

Very quickly and without any warning he grabs me to him and starts to pull up my T-shirt. He knows that I never wear a bra, even though I'm a big size. In a trice he's got my tits out and is sucking them. This drives me wild, but it's all rather sudden, even for me.

'Hold on, Jim,' I say. 'Give us a moment, love. I'm still a bit tired after an evening serving you lot.'

'What you need, my girl, is a nice rest,' he says. 'Come over here.' And he takes me to the garden swing that the kids play on. He undoes my skirt and lets it fall to the ground. 'Take your panties off, you sexy bitch,' he commands. Without even questioning it I do as he says. 'Right, now bend over the swing, with your stomach down, so your behind is towards me,' he orders.

I do as he says, lowering my poor belly on to the slightly damp seat of the swing. With my legs and feet off the ground he now swings me gently backwards and forwards. Every time I come back towards him he slides a finger into my wet cunt. In fact this is the only place he touches me at all as he pushes me off with his hand.

'Not much of a size for you, this, is it?' he asks. 'You need something a bit thicker.'

The next thing I'm aware of, he gives me a really big push and when my body comes back to meet his I feel my cunt smashing back on to his gigantic prick. I can't help screaming out, it's such a big bastard. He's gigantic and I'm quite relieved when he pushes me off him to make the swing go forward again. Trouble is, what goes forward must come back and I wait with anticipation at the thought of his giant prick waiting for me next time my body swings back to meet his.

Sure enough it slams into me again. The sheer depth of it is just like the first time.

'You're a sadistic bastard,' I say, gritting my teeth, but loving it. But he just pushes me forwards again to repeat the pleasure.

I'm getting a real taste for it myself now, and am about to come.

'Get on with it and make me come,' I cry out as he pushes me forwards for the fourth time.

With this he grabs my hips and keeps his prick in me rather than pushing me forward again. His thrusting sends shudders through me and I moan loudly as I come and come.

SOMEONE YOU KNOW BUT HAVEN'T HAD SEX WITH

This is a relatively straightforward fantasy type. Being involved with a current partner doesn't mean that others go away. They don't and they have to be dealt with somehow. Promiscuity, that is to say, doing something physical with anyone or everyone we find desirable, is unacceptable to most people, especially since AIDS made it dangerous.

Adultery in the mind is discussed on page 158. But whatever the moral argument on the matter, people will continue to have arousing fantasies about others to whom they are attracted, but with whom they have not had sex. In my view this is a highly successful way of dealing with the reality of one's own sexuality and that of others in a society that calls for monogamy, even if for many people reality means that the monogamy is serial (having a one-to-one relationship with one person after another).

LOVE MY NEIGHBOUR

My next-door neighbour is a real beauty. I take every opportunity to flirt with her in real life and would love to have sex with her.

My favourite fantasy is that one day she's out in her garden, kneeling down planting out some flowers. I look over the fence and see that her skirt is hitched up, showing her delicious thighs. I can see nearly up to her panties. I almost come at the thought of this alone on some occasions, but usually hold myself back for greater pleasures.

Taking my courage in both hands, I now scramble stealthily over the low fence and, creeping up behind her, kneel on the grass and slowly run my hands up her legs towards her panties. She doesn't move an inch, she just carries on with her planting as if nothing was happening. My hands rove all over her behind and I start to put my fingers into her panties to feel her vagina. It's wet and hot.

'I hope your hands are clean,' she remarks quietly, still without turning round. I'm taken aback because I didn't think she knew who it was. 'And I'd like something a bit meatier than your fingers while you're at it,' she says.

'Not out here,' I reply. And with that I pick her up and carry her into the garden shed.

I lie her carefully down on the potting table and deftly remove her skirt and panties.

'You spend so much time on your garden,' I say, 'I wonder if anyone pays as much attention to you.'

With that I pick up a half-full watering can from the floor and start to drip its contents teasingly over her pubic hair. I deliberately allow the drops to play right on to her clitoris, one tantalizing drop at a time. Soon she's obviously getting turned on.

'Have you got one of those things I see you using to put new plants in?' I enquire.

'You mean a dibber?' she asks.

'That's it,' I reply. 'Where is it?'

She motions to a shelf and lying there is the object I had in mind. I often watch her from my top window as she forces the thick, pointed wooden implement into the yielding ground before dropping in a small plant.

I take the dibber down from its resting place and blow the dust off. Parting her lips to insert the tool makes her open her legs wider in anticipation and she pushes herself towards the oncoming object in my hand. It's rather thick for her, but after some resistance she lets it in with a smile of delight.

'I'm ready for *you*, now,' she murmurs, after a while. 'Give me your dick.'

I take out my erect organ and, removing the wooden implement from her cunt, slide my prick into her wet, juicy hole.

'This is what you get for showing me your thighs, you little tease,' I cry, as I pound in and out of her and ejaculate.

She smiles a wicked smile that tells me this is what she'd planned all along.

SEX WITH AN UNSEEN PARTNER

If being irresistible largely removes the guilt associated with sex, having sex with someone unseen is even more effective for many people. I find this fantasy is most common in women, although men sometimes want to be taken over by an unseen woman. This need for males to be passive, or rather not to have to take the lead, is far more common than is generally thought. In so many spheres today – as friends, lovers, husbands, fathers and professionals – males are expected to shine. Many say they find this so wearing that they yearn for a sexual partner who will do gorgeous things to them unasked, and with no romantic or relationship price to pay.

'Unseen partner' fantasies answer these needs perfectly. The fantasists have things done to them and respond to their fantasy partner's wishes without question or hesitation, almost as if under an anaesthetic.

Many women have fantasies involving a male who has no face or head. This could be explained by asserting, as some women do, that they don't much mind who the man is, so long as he does exactly what they want – one in the eye for the romantic fiction brigade – or there could be more deep and important reasons.

I think that the faceless or headless man of many women's fantasies is an important male, perhaps even her father, whose identity would be too traumatic to cope with, even in the unconscious. Working with such women clinically, I often find that the identity of the man turns out to be someone significant from her past, often from her childhood. The implications of all this are unknown to the woman until we work through them in therapy.

Just as in dreams, symbols are often used in place of significant individuals in sexual fantasies. In both situations the symbolic individual or object protects the dreamer from openly confronting a difficult issue. I know it is a generalization, but in my experience the more up-front a woman is about her sexuality, the more she fantasizes about real individuals rather than faceless or unseen ones. In other words, such fantasies are often, but not always, a sign of an inhibited individual. As a woman becomes more able to deal with her sexuality in all its guises she begins to have real sex with real males and I know our therapy is succeeding.

A SATISFIED CUSTOMER

My best fantasy takes place in the lingerie department of a large store. I'm buying something really sexy to wear for our wedding anniversary. I spend quite a while choosing things and take them to the dressing-room to try them on.

As I stand there admiring myself in the mirror, I'm amazed and shocked to feel a pair of what are obviously male hands emerging around the curtains to touch me. They stroke me and caress me, running all over my breasts, which are looking wonderful and feeling great in a sexy new black lace number. Their owner runs his exploring fingers all over the soft mounds of flesh, stopping only a second or two to caress my nipples.

Soon, his hands are on my stomach and travelling down to my panties. He teases me with his fingers around the gusset, as if to go inside, but doesn't.

'Cover the mirror with your coat,' he orders in a whisper.

Still confused but quite excited by the whole prospect I throw my designer wool and cashmere coat over the free-standing mirror.

'Stay as you are and don't turn around,' he commands.

Before I know what's happening the curtain that separates the next cubicle area from mine slides apart and I'm aware that the man is right there behind me. Without a word he unhooks my bra and lets it fall to the ground. Next he gently but assertively removes my panties and tosses them on to the chair.

'Bend over and rest your hands on the chair,' he tells me.

I do what he says, still speechless and astonished at my own readiness for the adventure. He now comes up behind me and

Anonymity is always a popular theme. This woman's fantasy is that she will be brought to orgasm by her partner secretly when she is out to dinner with him one evening.

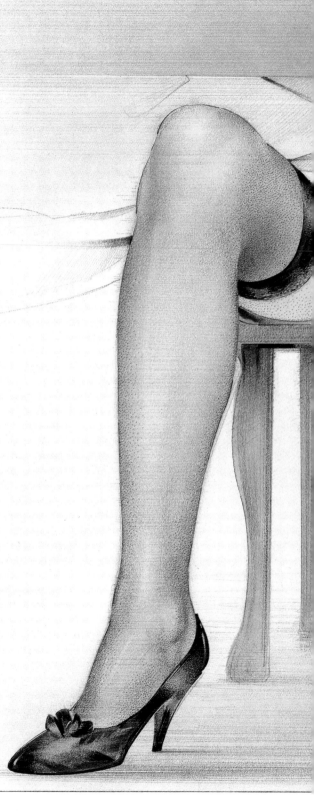

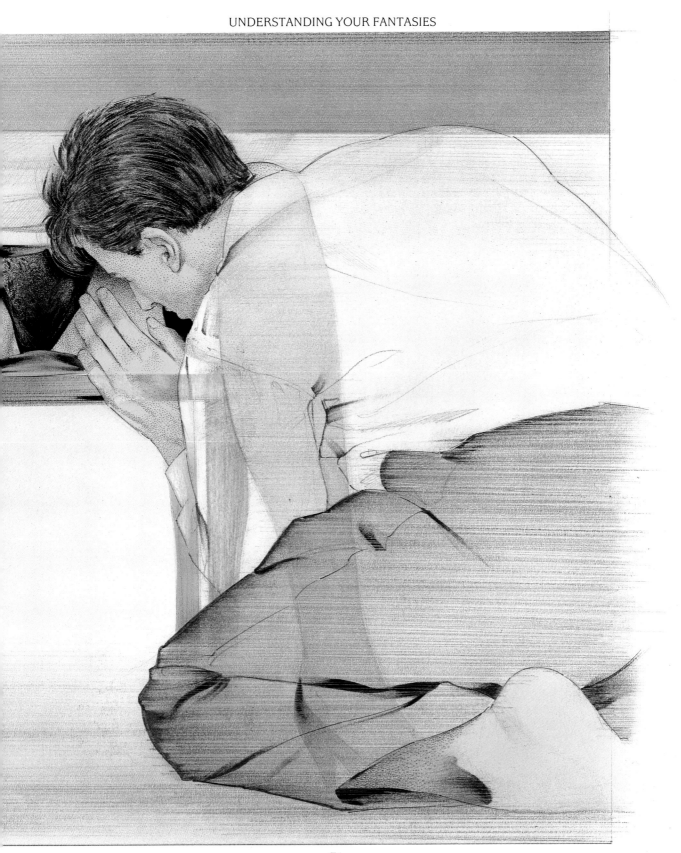

parts my feet so that I'm standing there with my fanny exposed to his gaze and exploring hands. He reaches round to grasp my breasts. He holds them firmly and squeezes them. I want to let out a yell but he whispers that unless I want to bring the whole game to an end I'd better keep quiet. I still don't know why, but I do as he says.

He kneads my nipples until they're quite sore, rolling them between finger and thumb, pulling them out from my breasts so that they're an inch or more long, then flicks them before holding the whole of my breast and mashing it hard.

'I expect you're quite hot by now,' he whispers in my ear.

I suddenly realize to my horror that he's the man who just directed me to the dressing-room. His hand now searches out my wet vagina and, before I can move a muscle, he has two fingers inside me, exploring my most intimate places. My feelings are beyond description as he slowly and systematically pushes his probing fingers into parts of my vagina that I didn't know existed. He caresses the front wall, too, which at first feels unfamiliar but soon becomes so exquisite that I think I'll die with the pleasure. My knees begin to tremble and I can hardly stand. Slowly and tantalizingly he works his magic on my insides.

When he takes his fingers out I can't bear it. I feel so empty, so yearning to be filled. Needless to say, I'm not kept waiting long. With a swift thrust, his penis is inside me and he's holding my hips to steady himself and prevent me from moving forward and away from his thick erection. He fucks me and fucks me so that I start to make little crying noises and know I will soon have to climax. He, realizing that this will make trouble for us both, bends down to the chair and, picking up my panties, gags me with them, to stifle the evidence of my arousal.

Now he's free to take me to the heights of ecstasy, which he does pretty expertly. Once he has ejaculated, he bends down and kisses my back tenderly.

'I hope the undies have the same effect on your husband,' he whispers, and is gone.

Anticipation can be half the fun in many sexual settings. She is preparing for a date with her new boyfriend, and day-dreams about him as she does so.

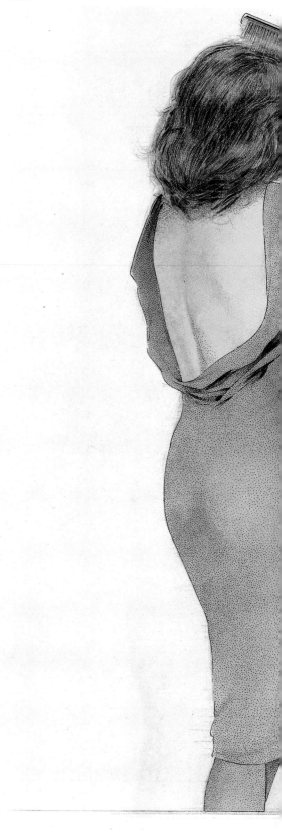

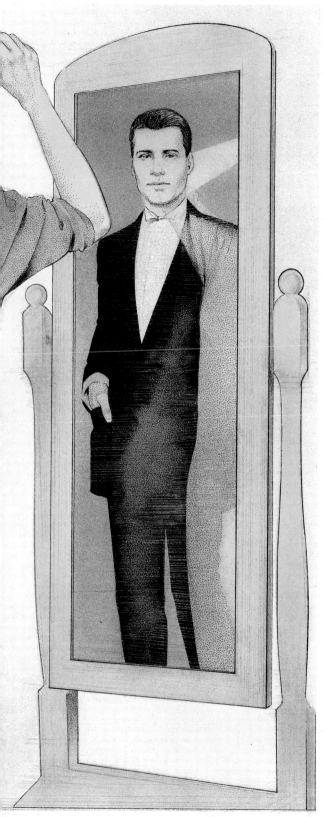

SEX WITH A STRANGER

Sex with someone you don't know often promises great rewards. In reality this sort of sex often works out rather badly, but in fantasies such practicalities are brushed aside in favour of the promise of the new, and the romantic joy of being so sexy and desired by another, completely unknown, person.

Sex with a familiar partner may well be fun, interesting and fulfilling, but many people are taunted by the suspicion that there must be more to sex. As a species, human females and males seem to be sexually adventurous. This lays the individual open to the seductive notion that the grass on the other side of the fence might just be greener. But how can individuals in a stable, one-to-one relationship, and worried about AIDS, herpes and the rest, hope to satisfy their yearnings for variety?

It can be seen from many other fantasies that this can be achieved in sexual reveries by experiencing the new with someone other than a current partner. In fantasies involving sex with a stranger this is taken yet one guilt-reducing step further by becoming involved in a short-lived flurry with someone unknown. Gone are the practicalities of a real relationship with all its restrictions and needs to show consideration. Gone the realities of having to become acquainted with someone in order to have true sexual intercourse (as opposed to copulation). The reward is pure, unadulterated sexual pleasure, unconditional and acceptable simply for what it is – a good lay.

With today's emphasis on togetherness, many men, especially, tell me of their efforts, in the bedroom and out of it, to please their woman. The New Man is under pressure to be empathic, sensitive, sensual, loving, a good dad, a thoughtful householder, an understanding boss or employee, and many other things. What an increasing number are saying is, 'How can I just have a really good fuck and not have to watch my step all the time?'

Sex-with-a-stranger fantasies allow just this. The only item on the agenda is lust. There is no prior business and there will be no future business. This is what is so arousing in such fantasies. It's sex for sex's sake, with no pretences and no price to pay.

Many women who have such fantasies say that only at these times do they feel able to be themselves. Some women find it hard to reveal their true sexuality to their loved man for fear that he will be unable to cope with it, might even turn away in disgust or might think them unacceptably pushy. 'If only he knew what I'm really like,' is the sort of thing I often hear.

Similarly, a man who might love his partner and get a lot out of making love with her will say that there are things he simply couldn't do with the beloved mother of his children. This is the sort of thinking at the heart of male fantasies of sex with prostitutes.

In sex-with-a-stranger fantasies, fears of sexually transmitted disease and unwanted pregnancies – which could plague such sexual adventures in real life – are dispensed with, and the whole episode revolves around uncluttered sexual pleasure. For many people of either sex such an abandonment to pleasure is rare in a one-to-one long-term relationship.

People feel they can let their hair down, be themselves, show off, experiment and generally be outrageous, in sex-with-a-stranger fantasies because they will never see the other person again. An added thrill in this kind of fantasy is that the stranger is a completely unknown entity sexually. Some women tell me that it is this slightly scary fear of the unknown, of what they might be required to do, added to the feeling of total abandonment, that so turns them on in the fantasy. Many complain that their love-making in real life is predictable and unadventurous, so it's hardly surprising that the completely unopened book of such fantasies lets their mind wander to sexual joys they couldn't indulge in real life.

Men might be seen as boring and unimaginative in many relationships, but women, according to many men, are frigid or inhibited, or simply 'won't do what I want'. For such men (and they are very numerous) a fantasy that involves a woman who just wants him and sex for itself can be such a holiday from reality that it makes the daily sexual drudgery of their lives bearable.

Angela, a highly intelligent and attractive woman in her late twenties, wrote this fantasy after a therapy session in which we had started to explore her feelings of boredom and exasperation with her well-meaning but sexually lacklustre husband. Like so many fantasies it had some basis in reality. She was, in fact, having her hall tiled at the time, as in her story:

UNEXPECTED ECSTASY

I'd been dressmaking and getting into a real stew about it when the doorbell rang. I was standing in complete 'at home' dishevelment, preoccupied with anger, because I'd been waiting for a long overdue visit from a man to tile my hall. What I actually got was better than that, I realized, as soon as I saw standing on the doorstep an intensely desirable being who could also tile a floor.

I could feel my eyes widen with pleasant surprise and I wondered if he noticed the tell-tale muscles move across my face. For a split second I thought I saw a mutual acknowledgement in him, but I put this thought to one side as I told myself to concentrate on the business in hand. After all, I might not be quite what he was expecting. I did look a mess. A tape measure hung around my neck, my frayed T-shirt was liberally decorated with pins and thread, half of it was tucked into my jeans, while the other half spilled over my belt. My hair was struggling out of a rather makeshift ponytail on to my bare, unmade-up face, with pale lips and eyelashes contrasting against my artificially acquired sun-tan. Traces of sleep were still etched into the texture of my skin.

He, on the other hand, was gorgeous. He was the type you never seem to see passing by in the course of day-to-day events, they just sort of appear. Once he had ascertained who I was, he introduced himself as Peter. We shook hands. I noticed in his voice the soft remnants of a North-of-England accent, to which I was particularly partial, and was struck by his air of warm, friendly self-assurance, which seemed to summon my attention.

I tried hard not to let him see my eyes looking over his body as we walked into the hall, but they furtively did so, awarding top marks in every category. He was tall, my favourite type, at least six feet two inches. That was good. Longish blond hair – I don't usually go for that, but it suited him. Great blue eyes. A figure that was athletic without being a cliché, I guessed he was too subtle for that; I knew he was strong and fit and knew he didn't have to prove it. Age? Probably around 30. Yum. Yum. I was practically licking my lips already.

I impressed myself with my cool, succinct briefing about the tiling and left him and his assistant to begin. I stayed for most of the day at the top of the house dressmaking, popping down only twice to check briefly on how things were coming along. Each time I was aware of myself, the young, vivacious mistress of the house, busily organizing, and aware too of how he affected me, the stirrings in my breasts each time I saw him. I noticed the way I moved, stood and talked in his presence, not affecting any unnatural postures, but I'd sensed that my body was doing its damnedest to make him notice me, even if my mind was far too respectable to join in.

I wasn't expecting him to arrive alone the next day. I'd already decided to work in the dining room, and continued to distress the paintwork of some drawers there, sitting cross-legged on the floor as he worked in the hall outside. My hair was once more struggling out of its ribbon and my lilac T-shirt tucked into jeans, again barely on my shoulders. I went upstairs to get a picture I'd intended for this room, to try to make the image of it more complete in my mind. Peter walked by as I held the picture out with both hands, squinting at the wall on which it would rest. He gave another approving nod and a quick smile, and carried on.

'Should the frame be black or white?' I thought to myself. 'It needs to be ornate, I think . . .'

Two hands pressed down on to my bare shoulders from behind me, tipping the last traces of T-shirt off on to my arms, and then slowly and firmly slid down on to my breasts. They held me there transfixed. Disbelief charged through my body. My mouth fell open, I gasped, but I didn't move. Neither of us moved for a moment. Then my shock began to dissipate and as it did so the hands began to stir.

Still clasping at my breasts, bit by bit the fingers relaxed their grip to explore the soft tissue. They sought out my now erect nipples, circling and pulling. I felt a deep breath escape my body, and the sound signalled a mouth to move against my neck and kiss; sweet succulent, nibbling kisses. I felt faint with pleasure. I was still holding the picture in my outstretched arms, frozen in the moment that he approached me, but my arms were getting weak. I came to enough to put the picture down, but before it came to rest on the sideboard a hand lifted it out of mine and put it on the floor against the wall.

I had to turn around and face this person who was controlling me, and as I did and saw his face, he wrenched the T-shirt from my torso, making it fall to my waist, leaving me naked. I kissed him with an overwhelming hunger, seeking out the pattern of his lips, moving my tongue into his mouth to find his. Our mouths joined in a frenzy of lust, his arms fell around my back and I felt my breasts press against him. My neck was aching from meeting his height and slowly I began to fall against the sideboard. He was almost catching me in slow motion, moving down to support my waist with one hand, caressing my nipple with the other.

I tugged the shirt from around his waist and pulled it free from his shorts. Frantically I ran my hands over his back, eagerly exploring flesh. He lifted the shirt up over his head and dropped it on the floor. Kneeling now, he stroked and massaged my breasts with both hands and kissed the side of my waist. I lowered my body, offering my breasts to his mouth. I felt the chill of his tongue run over my nipple, making it even more turgid than before, and I reached to unfasten the belt of my jeans. The noise of the metal buckle loosening made me quicken with anticipation and become aware of the throbbing pulse that was pounding in my swollen lips.

As his mouth worked on my breasts, my jeans fell to the ground and I shuffled them out of the way. We knelt together, flesh against flesh, kissing and exploring, at one moment tender, so tender, at another frenzied. Our eyes smiled when they met. I reached for the swollen erection threatening to burst out of his shorts and ran my hand up and down over the fabric. Then he lifted me up off the floor by my sides until I was lying on the sideboard with him bending over me. He kissed my mouth, my breasts, so many parts of me I could hardly take in the volley of exquisite sensations that his kisses created.

Then, a single action made me shriek with agonizing pleasure. His fingers delved under the fabric in between my legs, letting forth with them a torrent of moist liquid on to my lips and public hair. The pleasure was unbearable. Quickly he sank his fingers deep inside my cunt and spread the moisture over my clitoris, rubbing up and down repeatedly, running his hand all over hair and cunt until all I could feel was throbbing wetness everywhere. I wanted to explode. Two fingers went inside me, then three, pushing up and down, stretching me, making me ache for more, then back to my clitoris, skilfully demonstrating just how frantic he could make me feel.

I wanted to beg him to fuck me, to make his semen dispel some of the turmoil within me, but I refused to let him know just how vulnerable I was. It wasn't necessary in any case. I was on the brink of shouting out, writhing and groaning with unbearable, wet ecstasy, when he pulled down his shorts and, with a tug of his hand, freed his deliciously hard prick.

I just had time to see it before I felt him bury it in me, forcing my inner lips apart. I could feel it rubbing against the entire length and width of my cunt as we moved together off the edge of the sideboard, sweat now glistening between hands and skin as we caressed each other and fucked determinedly. As we rose and fell together I couldn't believe that two near strangers could be so devastatingly co-ordinated in bed – or even on the furniture – but we seemed to understand each other so well. The sexy ache of my vagina told me I was being well and truly screwed. And I loved every minute of it.

All I could see in my mind's eye was his magnificent cock rubbing against my insides, its friction making me want to split myself in two to receive more. I breathed deep, urgent breaths, barely conscious now as he lifted me up by the small of my back to push further. His breathing quickened, and for the first time I sensed his own pleasure as he approached orgasm. With steady, rhythmic thrusts, he spurted into me, cooling me, yet bringing a luxurious warmth at the same time.

It seeped out on to my lips and hair as he slowly withdrew, and, as he bent down to rest on me, my legs hung limply off the sideboard, leaving my exposed cunt dripping. He knew I hadn't come, though he didn't know how close I'd been, marooned on a delicious plateau almost from the beginning. He was going to make me come. I could sense his renewed determination and if anyone could do it, I knew it would be him.

Straightening himself up to look at me, his eyes assessed me with distant restraint. Now I was totally at his mercy. With the heel of his hand he rubbed the whole of my soaking vulva, pulling my lips apart, spreading our mingled cum to the far corners of my pubic hair. Still there was more moisture. With his fingers he dipped into my cunt and spread some of it over my nipples, tugging them lightly. I shuddered. I knew what was going to happen next and I braced myself.

He lowered his head in between my legs and I waited. Then, in one piercing movement, he sank his tongue into my cunt. I let out a little shriek, and then another as it rose and spread itself over my clitoris. It was like wet, warm velvet. I was ready now. He played with my nipples as his mouth took me further towards impending orgasm, licking me inside and out, slithering over my clitoris and then sinking deep into me again.

He took my clitoris into his mouth and played with it devotedly. I writhed with joy.

'Please God don't stop,' I cried.

I could see broken images of tongue, swollen clit and saturated cunt in my mind, all of them working to increase my pleasure. Suddenly my body joined in. Every muscle was coming together to share in this orgasm. His tongue deftly carried on as my back arched and I felt the pleasure seep into every vein. The world was going black. My body rose to meet the impending onslaught of climax. I felt a wave of joy contract throughout my body, like a giant swallow, and I became engulfed in the most consuming orgasm I've ever had, pulsating through me until I seemed to drown in pleasure.

SEX WITH TWO OR MORE PEOPLE

This is a topic recounted by both sexes, but probably more by men, who are brought up to be more sexually adventurous than women and to take more sexual risks. They're used to making things happen and to getting more of what society has to offer. This acquisition of goodies naturally includes women. Consequently, many men are aroused by the notion of having sex with more than one woman at once, although their reverie usually stops short of a true orgy, in which many couples make love with each other and everybody else.

Many males harbour conscious or unconscious fears about sexual performance, yet have only one woman to satisfy, so it's not too surprising that they have fantasies in which they pleasure several women at one session to lay these fears to rest. Clinical experience shows that the vast majority of such men would not and could not cope with such sexual demands if they were made in real life. The idea is so terrifying it can be dealt with only in fantasy. There is an additional thrill for some, when two or more of the women involved indulge in lesbian love-making.

Men who play around in real life say they want to do so against the secure background of their one-to-one relationship. This is why women complain that men want to have their cake and eat it. But this is exactly what most men do want: the security of their mother to come back to, as well as the fun and adventure of the world to go out to. In a sense, fantasizing about sex with two or more people epitomizes this desire.

Some men try to overcome these dilemmas in fantasy life by involving their wife in the fantasy sex games with others. According to such men, this involves her in their fantasy lives in a way that brings them closer together as a couple, furthers their one-to-one bond, and enhances their value to one another. In real life, swinging and swapping usually achieve exactly the opposite. Jealousy and hatred are never far away from such adventures, and long-term committed relationships usually suffer badly. In fantasy, such details are omitted and infidelity can appear to be sanctioned by the man's partner.

Sometimes – and this applies to both sexes – such a fantasy simply demonstrates the need to be seen as so sexy and attractive that two or more people can easily be accommodated; and to have more than enough sheer lust and attractiveness to please all comers. Pippa's fantasy is a good example of this:

MY DELIGHTFUL SANDWICH BREAK

In my fantasy I'm walking one day past a building site near where I work in London. As usual the men wolf-whistle at me and I must say I'm rather flattered. After all, I'm nearly 40 and have three kids, so to have all these lusty young men whistling at me is an ego trip.

Anyway, in my fantasy, as I walk along near the site I fall over some scaffolding that has been left lying around. I crash to the ground in a rather ungainly way, dropping all my shopping. Two of the guys rush to my aid and pick me up.

'Sorry,' one of them says. 'Shouldn't have left it there. Our boss would string us up by the heels if he knew.'

'Don't worry,' I say, 'I'll be all right.'

'You seem all right to me, darling,' quips the other guy. 'Sure your leg is OK?'

Before I know what's going on he lifts me bodily, takes me into their builders' hut and shuts the door. Laying me down on the enormous table spread with blueprints and plans, he starts to massage my leg where I hit it on the kerb.

'How does that feel?' he asks.

'It feels OK,' I reply, rather pathetically.

'How about me doing the other one, then?' asks his mate. And before I can say much he too has started to run his hard, powerful hands over my legs.

'I think I'll be all right now,' I say, panicking a bit as I begin to enjoy it.

'Be a shame to stop just when it seems to be doing some good,' says the first man. 'Lie back and enjoy it.'

By this time I'm getting quite horny, of course. The smell of their sweaty, strong bodies dressed only in jeans and vests is almost too much for me.

'Take her top off, Pete,' the first one says, 'I want to see her tits.'

The second guy does as he's told, even though I'm starting to struggle.

'No point making a fuss, love. No one will disturb us till tea break. We've got all the time in the world.'

My tank top off, and my breasts exposed to their gaze, I feel totally vulnerable – rather like a turkey at Christmas before everyone starts to tuck in. The second guy starts to suck my nipples, which really turns me on. He knows exactly the effect he's having. The other one, meanwhile, is taking off my panties and starting to finger my cunt. I'm so wet I'm ashamed of myself. Here I am, two complete strangers having their way with me, and I'm loving every moment of it. He stops feeling my cunt and looks up.

'Don't know about you, Pete, but I fancy a sandwich. How about you?'

'OK,' Pete says, and stops sucking my breasts.

Suddenly I'm disappointed. Surely the bastards wouldn't stop now and have time off for a snack, leaving me wet and ready to go?

Of course they wouldn't. Pete lies on the plan table on his back, his prick standing up

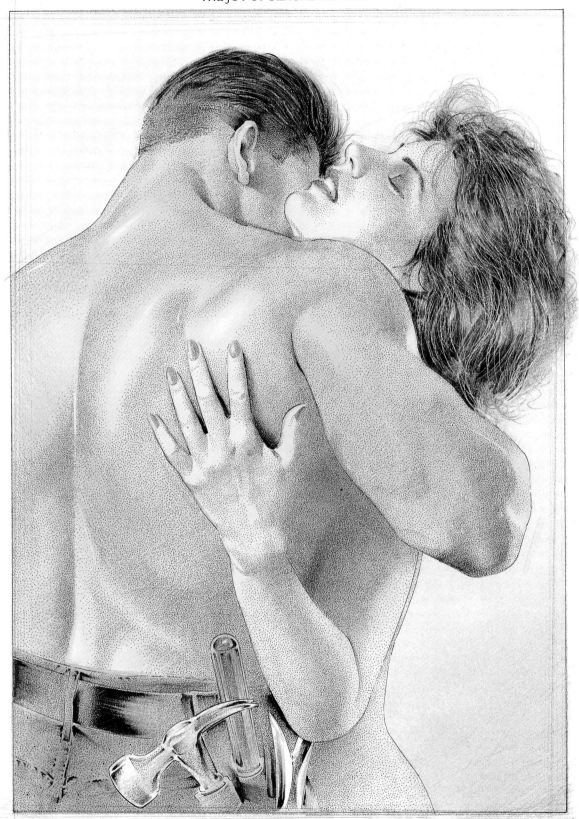

Big, beefy men, especially in fantasy, help some women feel tiny, helpless and very feminine. This can be just the trigger they need to make arousal possible or more enjoyable.

---

like one of the concrete pillars he builds. 'Get over me,' he orders.

I do as I'm told, scrambling over the plans so that I can straddle his enormous cock. Slowly I let myself down on to it, easing its full length into me. I'm so wet and open, it goes in without any trouble.

'Like that do we?' he asks, teasingly. My contented smile says more than any words. 'Lean forward on me, then, I want you to kiss me.' I do so and plunge my tongue into his mouth. In return I get an ironing board of a tongue that nearly chokes me.

But this is only the start. Pete's buddy is now on the table and coming up behind me, holding my hips. Slowly he plunges his prick into my anus, filling my whole pelvis with hot meat. I've never experienced anything like this before and can hardly breathe with the feeling of fullness. I normally like anal sex, but two pricks in me at once is too much. Suddenly I understand what sort of sandwich these guys had in mind. I am the filling.

With my mouth, cunt and behind full of sweaty male I'm not far from a shattering climax. As Pete grasps my tits and holds them tightly, his tongue thrusting in and out of my mouth, and his prick still inside me, his mate uses my behind in a way my husband has never done. I scream a muffled cry as he bucks and finally comes inside me. Pete and I come at the same time and my insides are awash with pleasure, wetness and pricks.

ORGIES

These are uncommon fantasies, even among men. Small-group sex, where the man is largely in control (*see* page 76), is rather different. In true orgies there's always a threat – albeit an unconscious one – that the man might become the hunted rather than the hunter. If this occurs at the hands of another man; or even if, during sex with a woman in a threesome, he comes into sexual or genital contact with another man, the whole event can go sour.

Homophobia, the fear heterosexual men have of the sexuality of other men being directed at them, is rife in Western society. A real man fucks, he doesn't get fucked. At a true orgy there's a serious danger that the proceedings could get out of control. This is why, in my view, I hardly ever hear men describing fantasies to do with orgies. Sometimes they've read about an orgy or seen something on a video or film that triggers the idea, but spontaneous orgy fantasies are pretty rare.

Peter's story is based on real swapping parties he ran in the late nineteen-sixties, but I'm sure that past reality has been somewhat embellished in his recollecting and retelling it when he masturbates:

MUSICAL SHARES

'Hi Peter,' says my best friend as we arrive at his Christmas party. 'Come on in. You're looking great, Miranda,' he says, admiring my wife, who looks brilliant that evening.

We go into the living-room where there are about ten other couples eating, drinking and dancing. 'Sorry we're late, Bill,' I say, as it's clear that the merrymaking has been going on for some time.

'Don't worry chum, you're here now, get yourself a drink. What will you have, Miranda?'

We're soon mixing with the others and everything is going well when Bill announces that there's going to be a game. Bill is well known for his sense of fun, so we all heave a sigh and settle down to see what the game will be.

'I'm going to play some music for dancing, and when it stops I want each person to take a piece of clothing off his or her partner, and then change partners for the next dance. Everyone got it?'

We certainly have, but I'm not at all sure if we like it. Miranda and I have run swinging parties in the past, but we've put all that behind us. We had no idea Bill was into this, but after a quick chat we decide to go through with it. After all, if the game gets too heavy, we argue, we could cut out, make our excuses and leave. Bill would understand.

So Bill starts up the music and Miranda and I dance together. He lets it run for quite a few minutes so that we almost forget about the game. When it stops, she takes off my necktie and I take off her bracelet.

We smile at each other and change partners as the music stops.

This continues for some time until the whole mood starts to hot up. Miranda is now down to her bra and panties and the man she's dancing with has only his shirt on. I organize it so that I get close to her at the next change of partners and, after removing her bra, I take her in my arms and dance with her. She looks stunning. I'm so proud of her. She has a better figure than most of the other women. She seems so confident, having a great time.

'Sure you want to go through with this, darling?' I ask. 'We can always leave.'

'I'm loving every minute of it,' she replies. 'We'll see who chickens out first: Bill and his friends, or us.'

I give her a squeeze. 'What a woman,' I think to myself. 'She's got more guts than I have.'

Although this theme is unpopular with men, quite a few women say that they like the idea of being the centre of sexual attention in a kind of 'orgy'.

The music changes again and most people are now completely naked, dancing cheek to cheek, chest to boobs. Erections abound and it's clear that before long people will be wanting to do something about them.

'Right,' says Bill, stopping the music. 'Now we're all acquainted I want each woman to get a ruler from the table over there and find out how long her partner's cock is. The winner gets a prize.'

The sight that follows is something else: ten women all on their hands and knees, measuring the penis of a man they hadn't even met until a couple of hours before.

'Right, then. Anyone over 6 inches?' A show

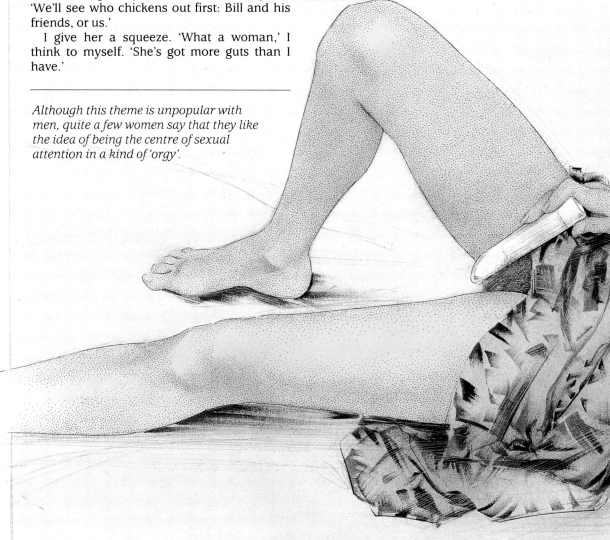

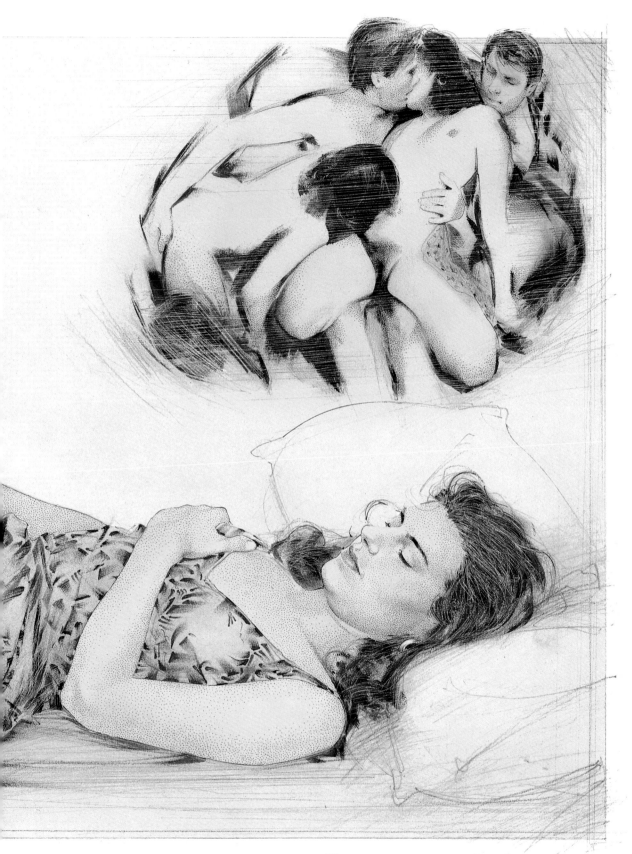

of hands. 'Over 9 inches?' Two ladies keep their hands up. 'Tell me how long, Jenny.'

'Nearly 11,' she calls across the room proudly, as if it were her regular partner.

'Anyone beat that?' No one could.

'Come on over here, big boy,' he says to the winner, 'and collect your prize.' With that he takes the lucky man over to the curtain that separates the living-room from the dining area and with a flourish, draws it aside. There, behind the curtain, lying on the dining-room table dressed only in a dab of Chanel and her best necklace, is Bill's 30-year-old second wife, Christine.

'Give the lucky winner his prize then, Chris,' Bill whoops.

She, delighted, open her legs and draws the fortunate, if embarrassed, man towards her. He rises to the challenge and plunges straight into her with his full 11 inches. This gives her more than she bargained for, because she catches her breath and whimpers a little. She soon starts to enjoy herself, though, and as we all watch and cheer him on, he brings her to an orgasm with his powerful thrusting.

As you can imagine, it's no time at all before the rest of us are doing the same with whoever is available. But the greatest turn on of all, and what makes me come like mad when I use this fantasy, is looking across to see Bill pumping his cock in and out of Miranda as she leans her graceful arms against the sofa.

As she wriggles her gorgeous little ass and pushes it out to meet his oncoming organ I come and come, almost oblivious to the woman who's sucking me.

SADO-MASOCHISTIC THEMES

This is a highly complex and researched subject. Whole books have been written about each half — sadism and masochism — and there are numerous psychoanalytical interpretations that try to explain why people find the inflicting and suffering of physical pain sexually exciting, in fact or fantasy.

Strictly speaking, sadism is defined as the obtaining of sexual pleasure or orgasm by inflicting pain on another. Masochism is a condition in which the individual who is the subject of the pain becomes sexually aroused, perhaps to orgasm.

It is often said that males are more likely to be sadistic, and females, masochistic. Many distinguished analysts claim that females are intrinsically masochistic: seeking pain and humiliation; demonstrating a willingness to suffer at the hands of males; and needing to be sexually submissive. I don't agree with this. The view is naïve and doesn't take account of the fact that most people, male and female, have at least some sadistic and masochistic traits, however symbolic. It's also essential to bear in mind that it can often be hard, even for an expert, to tell which is really the sexual turn on at any one time for any one individual.

I shall deal with quite a few sado-masochistic (SM) sub-themes in this part of the book, because they all have common origins, intermingle with one another in people's fantasies, and are popular. For example, although most women don't have fantasies that involve suffering pain, countless millions of women fantasize every day about being 'raped', humiliated, dominated or otherwise having things done to them sexually. In the most profound sense I call this 'masochistic'; just as the male equivalents are termed 'sadistic'.

In sado-masochism, as in all other sexual tastes, it's a brave individual who would care to draw the line between normal, playful SM games in fact or fantasy, and the true sado-masochism of the pervert. There are no rigid boundaries.

This becomes even more confusing because although there are people who need real SM activities, in order to become aroused at all, many millions of others would never do such things in reality, yet can become aroused only if they do them in their fantasies. How perverted is such an otherwise normal individual? Probably not at all. Such people simply find that certain themes arouse them best, just as others who have non-SM fantasies do.

In broad terms it could be said that the majority of female sexual fantasies are mainly passive. That is, the fantasist is having things done to her. The advantage of such fantasies to the woman who is heavily burdened with sex guilt is that they absolve her from any responsibility for the resulting sexual pleasure. The man does everything and she is simply the innocent, yet desirable, object. That this sort of masochistic fantasy is so commonplace shows just how large a proportion of the female population in the West is still plagued by guilt about sex.

Contrary to the suggestion implicit in this observation, women are not wholly or largely masochistic. All the childhood influences that create sadistic tendencies in men also create sadistic tendencies in women. As I work with women I notice that they sometimes unconsciously project their sadism on to their men, so that they can act it out for them and thereby sanitize it. The same happens the other way around, when men project their masochistic needs on to their women, who oblige them by acting them out.

Some women are so unconsciously angry with their parents, usually their mothers, that they become what is called passive/aggressive. They appear to be nice, submissive, yielding and so on, but not very far down they're terribly angry at accumulated hurts from childhood or beyond. This unconscious aggression is then expressed by a woman's partner in sexual games, or by the woman herself in her SM fantasies.

For example, a woman who has fantasies of having her breasts hurt is often unconsciously acting out her hatred of her own mother. In this sense adult women, because they have ready access to the same objects that caused such early and primitive psychic pain in infancy, can all the more easily act out their hatred of the 'bad breast' that was represented by their mother. I feel that women's generally rather negative feelings toward their breasts (one study found that only a quarter of women were truly satisfied with their breasts) are further proof of all this.

The same study of 300 women of all ages showed that twice as many men squeezed their partner's breasts during love-making as wanted it. A common complaint from women is that their men tend to be too rough too soon with their breasts during foreplay. Some women do like having their breasts squeezed, even quite hard, during sex but the study found that half as many women again enjoyed squeezing their own breasts during masturbation as enjoyed having them squeezed by their man when making love.

What this all says about the desire both sexes seem to have to inflict some sort of pain on the female breast is confusing. What is interesting is that there seems to be no commonly experienced counterpart in which either sex does the same to the male genitals.

Other women – and I think they are numerous – wish unconsciously to confirm the cultural position of women in general and of themselves in particular. By having masochistic fantasies they maintain themselves where they 'ought to be' in the scheme of things, according to their own unconscious model. As I discuss later (*see* page 32) many women are perpetually guilty about something. It's often sex, but it extends way beyond this to many other areas of life. This guilt makes them feel, unwittingly, that they deserve to be punished for not being what they should be, in or out of bed. Such a need for punishment surfaces sometimes as masochistic fantasies, which may or may not be acted out in real-life sex games.

As you can see, much of the hidden agenda that produces masochistic fantasies is very old in psychological terms. In fact, I think SM fantasies are some of the most primitive, dating back, as they do, to very early in infancy.

Tiny babies quickly learn that their mothers can't be everything for them exactly when they desire it. Omnipotent infants want what they want when they want it, but such a system is bound to fail because no mother can possibly spend her entire life servicing her baby. When she does not answer her baby's needs, anger and frustration, and then hatred, may well up in the baby. Unfortunately babies can't hate their mothers too much, or indeed show their anger and frustration too much, because to do so might mean that even fewer of their needs would be answered and they might even be abandoned altogether. So babies begin to turn some of this anger inward, where it feels safe – if painful.

But when babies do this, they still experience a combination of love and hatred for their mothers, and this ambivalence is the start of SM fantasies. Some start manifesting themselves during infancy. How many mothers have experienced a furious baby biting a nipple during breast-feeding? Most people have noticed how angry a toddler can get when crossed. Such expressions of fury are especially common in those babies whose needs are often left unmet, or whose mother leaves them for long periods, so that they become lonely, frustrated, bitter and hateful. Such behaviour by the mother leads, in my view, to a baby who builds up hatred against her, yet it is hatred that can't be expressed openly for fear of the ultimate loss: the loss of the mother.

However well all this is masked at the time, it often reveals itself in later life as fantasy material. It's no accident that so many male sadistic fantasies focus on hurting women's breasts. Very extreme examples of such fantasies involve cutting off the woman's breast, or some sort of symbolic equivalent. A man who harbours such fantasies was undoubtedly murderously furious at the breast in infancy, perhaps because he was denied what he wanted. Now he needs somehow symbolically to punish all women for it.

Many inhibited men find that they need sexual enhancers if they're to function. Some of the most effective of these involve deep, unconscious material that enables them to act out, if only in fantasy, what they really want to be doing to a woman. If in real life a man's mother was restrictive or even punishing towards him sexually, he can, by symbolically punishing his fantasy woman, get back at his mother, albeit in a roundabout way. After all, many such men tell me, if women see sex as so unacceptable and awful (as their mother did), surely they will need to be forced to do it, or to be punished for their interest in it.

Childhood experiences make some individuals of either sex link sexual arousal with pain and humiliation. How this occurs is often not clear in any one case, but if, for example, a loved parent beats a child and even perhaps says this is because he or she loves the child, it's not hard to see how such a child could come to think of physical punishment as something that people who love one another mete out. For an individual who has been made anxious about sex during childhood – and this amounts to millions – focusing on the pain can take the mind off the anxiety caused by sexual arousal. By denying it in this way, the individual can then enjoy the sex.

TYING-UP FANTASIES

Being tied up or tying someone up are fairly common fantasies. Perhaps more women enjoy the former and more men the latter. Whenever people tell me that they like to tie up their partner, I always reflect to them that I think they really mean 'tie *down* their partner'. After careful consideration, such people often remember a childhood characterized by the absence of key loved ones, especially a mother. Experiences in early infancy of Mother

not being there may lead to adults who seek to ensure that their lovers stay there for them.

Some men say that they want to tie down their partner for sex so that she will have to accept her own sexuality. Many tell me of partners, who are otherwise somewhat inhibited, becoming highly aroused when made to have sex in this way: they have to accept their own sexuality because they can't do anything else.

Most people, like Tony in the next fantasy, use tying-up games in fact or fantasy to drive their partner wild with teasing before releasing him or her for really exciting sex. Tony uses his wife's immobility and helplessness to get to what he really wants – her breasts. In real life Tony was hardly breast-fed at all, because his mother was severely affected by post-natal depression and was scarcely available for him for some months.

BOUND TO PLEASE

This fantasy of mine is a real winner. I share it with my wife sometimes when we're both turned on. It starts off with me taking her to a sophisticated sex club, like those you hear about in Holland or Germany. She's willing, of course, because she's so sexy, but she doesn't know what she's letting herself in for.

When we arrive she's taken off by a very attractive female dressed in leather gear and I'm taken by a hostess to the bar to relax while I watch other couples doing the most outrageous things. Soon it will be our turn.

Within a few minutes the hostess brings my wife back dressed only in a G-string, with a thick leather-studded collar around her neck. There are soft leather cuffs around her ankles and wrists. She looks so sexy that sometimes I ejaculate at this point of the fantasy if I'm masturbating alone.

Anyway, back to the fantasy. The hostess asks me if I'd like to try out a new gadget they've just installed for women with large breasts, like my wife's. I eagerly agree, though I see my wife's face tense up as she wonders what on earth I'm getting her into.

The hostess leads us both to the stage area, where several couples are sitting around

This is a favourite fantasy, under various guises, of both sexes. The bonds tying her hands are more symbolic than real, but what matters is the exchange of power.

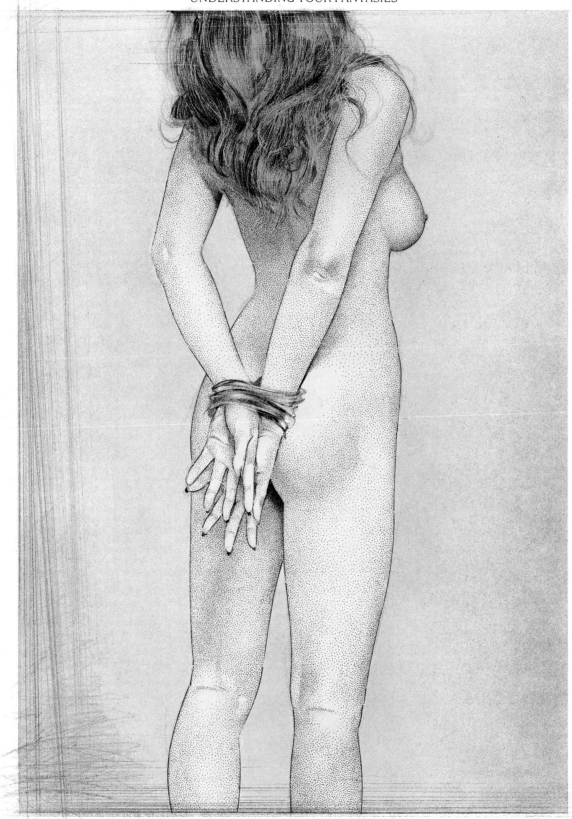

drinking and waiting for the next part of the show. From the ceiling she lowers a large hammock-like structure made of stout canvas. She tells my wife to get on it and then crosses to me. 'It's up to you now,' she says, and walks off.

I soon get the hang of the thing. There are two holes in the top end of the canvas, and clips at each corner near the supporting ropes. I get my wife to lie on the hammock face down and fix her wrist and ankle cuffs firmly to the corners of the hammock. I then raise the whole thing so that it comes to rest at about eye level and, reaching up, find her breasts and draw them out through the holes in the canvas.

She's now left suspended there in the air, totally immobile, her arms and legs wide apart, and all her body hidden except for her breasts, which fall out of the holes and are completely exposed, so that I can do what I want with them.

I start to play with her nipples and to squeeze her tits the way I like. She writhes in protest, but can't escape. Before long other people come up from the audience and play with her breasts. Women come up and suck them.

When my wife is really aroused the hostess returns with a riding crop and deftly swishes it across her body, while another woman sucks her nipples. This brings forth a stifled cry from my wife, who's obviously loving it, but in any case has no option but to go along with it. After a few minutes of this the whole hammock starts to writhe and buck as my wife lets out a deep, throaty moan. As she climaxes the audience gives a cheer.

Fantasies of being tied up have their roots in guilt (*see* page 32). Like so many other fantasies of its type, this one is much less passive than at first appears. After all, it takes two to play all these SM games and the partner who does the tying-up is every bit as involved in the unconscious games as the one who's tied. Unless the game in real life involves true coercion – and this is unusual – looking at the situation analytically, the woman who's tied might just as well be tying herself up.

Paula's fantasy is a good example of this. Like many, it also contains other elements. She's quite an inhibited woman, who not only needs to be tied up (in her fantasy) to become really excited but also to accept her desire for men other than her husband. It all ends well, with her having sex only with him; but early in the story it looks as though a gang-bang is on her unconscious agenda.

FAIR GAME

I love to fantasize about my partner tying me up to have sex. Sometimes I make it really simple. He just puts me down on the bed and ties my hands behind my back to make me completely unable to resist.

On other occasions, when I'm feeling horny and have lots of time, I use an even better fantasy. It involves my husband inviting some friends round to play poker one evening. They all have a few drinks and by the end of the evening are pretty drunk, but not at all disorderly. I come in from another room to find them talking about me and the way I like being tied up for sex.

'Perhaps we should help you, Andy.'

Another chips in, 'I expect she takes a bit of handling. She looks a spirited filly to me.' With that, Bob, who's speaking, gets up and grabs me firmly.

I struggle to resist because the joke's gone far enough. But it soon becomes clear that they're not joking – they really do intend to tie me up.

Andy, rather than coming to my rescue, is all for it. 'I'll get the ropes,' he volunteers.

The others come over to me and hold me to stop me from escaping. When Andy returns, each takes a rope and they start to tie my ankles and wrists.

'What shall we tie her to, Andy?' one asks excitedly.

'Bring her up to our bedroom,' he replies, 'I think you'll like what you see.'

'God, I see what you mean,' exclaims Bob when he sees our four-poster bed.

In seconds they've taken me to the bed, stood me up at one end and secured me firmly to the posts. My hands are immobilized at the top of each post and my feet securely tied to the bottom.

'Right,' says the one who's taking the initiative. 'Take turns now. One at a time, remove a piece of clothing. Fred, you can go first.'

Fred, an old friend of my husband, can hardly believe his luck. I know he's been turned on by me for years and has wanted to get his hands on me ever since we first met. Looking rather nervous and casting a furtive eye toward Andy, he steps over to me and unbuttons my blouse slowly. 'I won't be able to get this off with her arms up,' he says, but he still takes great pleasure in undoing it, pulling it out of my skirt and taking it off my shoulders.

'That's enough, Fred. My turn next.'

The second man now takes his place in front of me and, looking me directly in the eyes, reaches behind my back and unhooks my bra. 'Got any scissors in your bathroom, Andy?' he asks.

Andy goes to get the ones I use to cut his hair.

'Great,' he says, and confidently snips through my bra straps so that he can remove the whole thing. This he does with a flourish, to reveal my swollen breasts and erect nipples. 'I think we're having the desired effect on the lady, don't you, guys?'

They all nod in approval.

'Me next,' says Neil, my husband's best friend. He knows he can't get my skirt off because my legs are wide apart, so he tucks it up into its waistband, revealing my panties.

'Thank God I've got good ones on,' I think to myself. They're pretty bikini briefs with only tiny strings at the sides to hold them up.

'I think it's my turn with the scissors now,' he says as he cuts through the strings, and the panties fall to the ground between my legs.

There's only one more man left now, apart from my husband, and I have nothing left on to remove. He starts to complain about this, but Bob isn't going to leave him disappointed.

'As you've waited till last, you deserve something really nice. Do what you want with her – she won't mind.'

The last guy makes for me and I wonder what he'll do. He runs his hands over my tense breasts, their nipples ache with desire to be touched. After caressing them for a few seconds, he strokes my stomach and runs his hands around my behind, holding it sexily and stroking it just the way I like. In a few seconds he's down between my legs, fingering my labia and stroking my clitoris until I'm nearly ready to come.

'That's enough,' Bob interrupts. 'She's all yours now, Andy. We'll be off. See you at the club on Friday.'

With that they all leave the room without a backward glance.

Andy comes over to me and tells me that I'm the sexiest whore he's ever had the pleasure to fuck. He tweaks my nipples in my favourite way, rolls them and pulls them till I can bear it no more, then expertly works me to a climax with his fingers in and around my cunt. I come time and again, the orgasms rippling over my jerking body in waves. It seems like minutes before he stops, unties me and I fall on to the bed, exhausted.

PHYSICAL PAIN

Hurting and being hurt may or may not be involved in the restraint-type fantasies described above. Ben's fantasy started with a particular incident that he can consciously remember. I think this is an important example, because it shows how an individual can have an apparently normal and loving upbringing, yet be affected by a particular event in later life that creates a valuable basis for a fantasy. As a therapist, I usually find that the reason such an apparently isolated story takes root as a useful fantasy has much to do with unconscious matters that sometimes come to light in the course of the therapy.

THE PLEASURE OF PAIN

I know where and when my best fantasy originated. When I was about 14 I used to go to a barber's shop that had all kinds of magazines for the customers. One day I read this story about a soldier being caught in the jungle and tortured to give the whereabouts of his pals. When he wouldn't talk, they stripped him and started to squeeze his balls in a gadget that screwed down to clamp the balls between two flat surfaces, a bit like a thumb screw. He yelled in agony, but wouldn't give his friends away. His torturers continued to turn the screw until he could bear no more and lost consciousness.

My fantasy is that my girlfriend, who's really very gentle and sweet, will squeeze my balls very hard as I masturbate. I've tried doing this myself, but can't get enough pressure on my balls. In the fantasy she holds my balls, one in each hand, while she sits facing me between my open legs. I masturbate and ask her to squeeze me harder and harder until I ejaculate. This fantasy never fails to turn me on even when I'm not feeling horny. It gives me an erection to think about it.

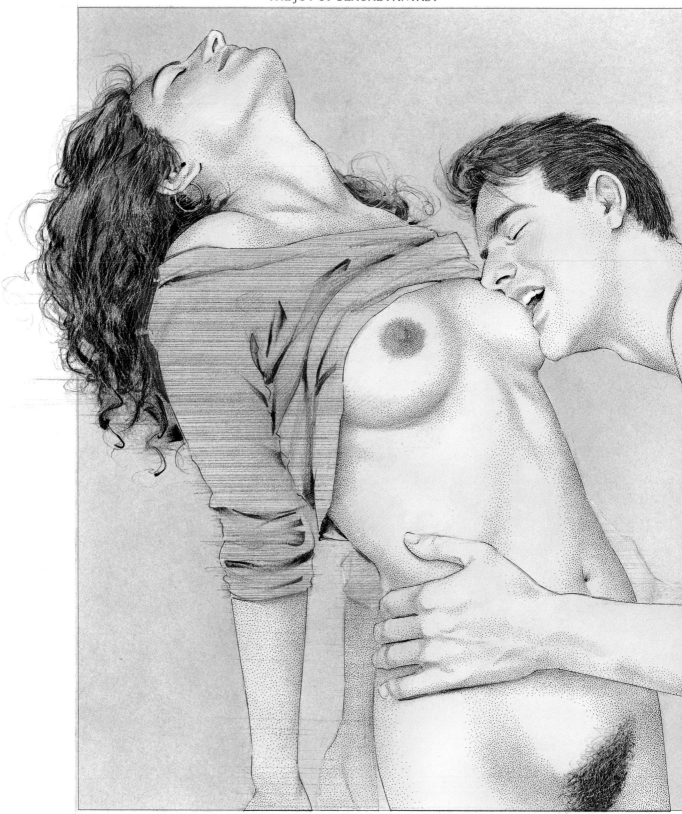

Many SM sessions, both in fact and fantasy, take on a highly ritualized tone, akin to old, pagan, black magic ceremonies. It's as though the events have the effect of a kind of sexual talisman, so it's essential that in the fantasy the players replicate exactly the right scenario every time the fantasy is used. Every minute detail of the SM theme is important and can't be changed if the imagined event is to have its best effect.

In a way, this ritual frees the individual to indulge in a quasi-spiritual experience that seems to make sense of what would otherwise be random events. Those who use SM activities in fact or fantasy sometimes talk of the transcendent power they endow. In a sense, SM fantasies are like adult fairy tales; and like such stories told to children, their predictability has an almost mystical power.

I have shortened Phillip's fantasy. The unedited version includes minute details of every fraction of the story. Once again, the pain is mainly inflicted on the woman's breasts. But before looking at Phillip's story, consider for a moment the fact that for much of their lives together, perfectly normal and ordinary couples play sex games that have sadistic or masochistic elements. The arousing love bite, the playful smack on the behind and the squeezing of nipples at orgasm are just a few examples of what most people would consider normal, everyday love play. In fantasy people who enjoy such things can let themselves go further.

Although I have suggested that there are usually psychological explanations for most fantasies, certain SM pursuits clearly have a biological background. I say this because some female animals ovulate only if bitten by their mate. While it's clear that women ovulate every month regardless of whether sexual intercourse took place, it's also true that a woman who is scared, perhaps during a rape, can ovulate even though it's not the correct time of her cycle. In this sense she is behaving like certain animals. This was discovered by analyzing the pregnancies resulting from rapes. Many of the women could not have been ovulating under normal circumstances, yet they became pregnant.

So perhaps some level of pain or fear is somehow intrinsic to female sexual functioning, at whatever primeval level.

TITILLATING TORTURE

My wife and I play sexy games that involve giving her pain as she climaxes. This isn't just a fantasy. She really does like her nipples squeezed firmly when we make love. But in my fantasy I go just that bit further to do things I'd like to do but haven't yet had the courage to ask her.

In my best fantasy I get my wife really aroused in the ways that she likes and then, when I put her on the bed, I take out some clips from my drawer and put one on each nipple. At first she says she finds them pleasantly tight, but as I arouse her more and her breasts swell, she asks me to take them off because they're hurting. I refuse and tell her that if she doesn't keep quiet I'll gag her. She begins to writhe and moan and as she does so I then go down on her and lick her pussy and clitoris to bring her off. As she gets even more aroused she can't bear the nipple pain any more, so I tie a wide belt made of soft material around her head to gag her.

Now I'm free to continue stimulating her in any way I wish. The clips on her nipples are really tight now and she can hardly bear it. I know it's time for her to come, so I bring her off quickly. She screams with the combination of the clips and the climax, and her abandoned cries make me ejaculate. I come all over her belly and, as I do so, I take the clips off her tits. This produces a surge of pain that's even worse than when they were on, and she yells uncontrollably as I shoot all over her chest.

Although some people's fantasies involve real pain and true sadism, most individuals settle for more symbolic pain as an extension of their love play. Many women, for example, say that they like their nipples squeezed or gently bitten as they climax.

BEING FORCED

Being forced to do something is a very common female fantasy. Into this category come 'rape' fantasies. I put the word in quotation

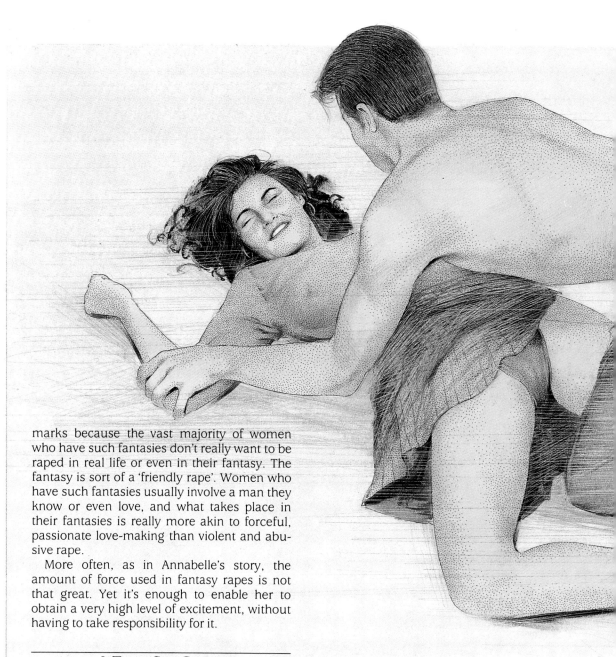

marks because the vast majority of women who have such fantasies don't really want to be raped in real life or even in their fantasy. The fantasy is sort of a 'friendly rape'. Women who have such fantasies usually involve a man they know or even love, and what takes place in their fantasies is really more akin to forceful, passionate love-making than violent and abusive rape.

More often, as in Annabelle's story, the amount of force used in fantasy rapes is not that great. Yet it's enough to enable her to obtain a very high level of excitement, without having to take responsibility for it.

A TRUE SEX SLAVE

I have lots of fantasies, but if I really want to get turned on I think of my Arabian harem one. In this I'm part of the harem of a very rich Arab prince. I know that of all his women he likes me best. He tries out all his favourite sex games with me first before the others and I consider it a great honour. I'm very sexy and able to take anything he makes me do, but it's a sort of battle of sexual wills as to who will get the better of whom.

Fantasies of 'rape' are popular with women and probably always will be. The owner relinquishes responsibility for her arousal as the man of her dreams overpowers her and makes her submit.

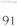

One day, the Prince sends a messenger to tell me to go to the arena where he holds his horse shows. He has some of the most fabulous horses in the world, worth millions.

In the next scene I'm in a room near the arena. I'm dressed only in an almost see-through, flowing white robe. The Prince motions to an underling to bring over a large case. He opens it up and inside is a range of dildoes, some as small as a finger and one so large it's about 3 inches across. Each is exquisitely carved in ivory and has a large, bulbous head and a flattened bottom under a large scrotum.

Without saying a word, the Prince comes over to me and gently makes me bend double. 'Touch your toes,' he bids.

I do so, of course, without question.

'The skirt,' he barks to his underling, who crosses over to me and lifts my robe up so that it rests over my back. 'The legs,' he hisses, and the underling parts my legs by pushing my feet apart as wide as they'll go.

Placing the case of dildoes in front of my gaze on a wide couch, the Prince now selects a medium-sized one and dips it in some sort of gooey liquid. 'Try this,' he orders.

The underling now gets behind me while the Prince sits on the sofa so that he can see my expression as the servant inserts it into my vagina. Although it's quite large it slides in easily.

'Much too small,' sneers the Prince. 'Take this one.' He selects a phallus twice the thickness of the previous one, but still nowhere near the biggest in the case. I know this will be a lot harder to take, so I close my eyes in anticipation of the pain.

'Open your eyes. I want to see them,' the Prince orders.

I do so and look pleadingly at him as his minion thrusts the larger dildo into me.

'Better,' says the Prince. 'Now we'll really get down to business.' So saying, he takes the second largest organ. It's a monster that I fear will split me open. I make to stand up.

'Hold her,' he yells to two other men who are watching. They hold my body over and cruelly force my legs open.

The feelings of fullness that follow are almost too much to bear. The large dildo bites into my insides, forcing the walls of my cunt apart and hitting my cervix deep inside. I screw up my eyes, not caring now whether the Prince is angry.

'I think she's ready now for her riding lesson,' he says, as he selects the largest dildo from the case. Handing it to the underling, he tells me to stand up.

As I do so I see some men bring in a priceless white stallion from the Prince's stable. It's such a handsome beast I can hardly believe it. It wears a saddle but no stirrups. The Prince knows I like riding; in fact sometimes we go riding together. To my amazement, the underling now goes over to the horse's saddle and screws the giant dildo on to it so that it stands up vertically, jutting high into the air.

'Mount her,' the Prince orders quietly.

Two men come over to me, remove my dress and take me to the horse. They lift me on its back and I grasp both arms around its neck in horror as I see what's about to happen.

One of them holds me in position over the dildo and the other guides its head into position under me. I grip the sides of the beast with my thighs, trying desperately hard not to let myself down on to the giant penis, which I know will tear me apart.

The Prince comes alongside the horse and gives it a sharp slap on the flank. The beast walks off toward the arena and I begin to lose my grip. A word of command from the Prince and the horse breaks into a trot, thrusting its wide, muscular back into the air rythmically as it circles the arena.

By now my legs have become so tired I can stand it no more and, as the animal starts to canter, the dildo shoots up into my cunt. The feeling of fullness almost makes me lose consciousness, but I hang on to the animal's neck. A further order, and it starts to gallop. The dildo is now thrashing in and out of me as I shoot around the track of the arena, the watching crowd obviously delighted at the spectacle.

By this stage I'm lost in oblivion as my cunt is pounded by the massive dildo. This makes me have orgasm after orgasm, in both the fantasy and real life.

Forcing someone to do something can include the simplest of normal sexual activities, such as here in Len's fantasy, or it can become much more sinister, verging on the perverted, if the partner is forced to do outrageous things. As with all the fantasy material I discuss in this part of the book, I have drawn a line at frankly perverted or psychiatrically disturbed material, which has a place only in a textbook for sexual physicians.

CRIME OF PASSION

In real life my girlfriend is a tease. She leads me on, then either cries off sex altogether, or makes me beg her for it. My fantasy is that one day, when she's been leading me on but not letting me have sex with her, I just throw her down on the bed and make her have sex. She struggles a lot but I force her legs apart viciously and tear her panties off.

She protests, but is obviously very excited by it all because she's so wet between her legs when I get my prick into her. I like to hear her yell as I push it in really deeply.

MALE SUBMISSION AND PASSIVITY

Males can be masochistic, passive, or submissive, too. An inhibited male can be so ashamed of his own interest in sex, which he has been taught is naughty and sinful, that he punishes himself by bearing the brunt of sexual pain at the hands of his real-life or fantasy lover. In the sadistic version of this he punishes the female for arousing *his* interest in sex.

The whole subject of male submission and passivity is a fascinating one and one which is being increasingly studied. It has been estimated that about 50 million Americans indulge in some sort of heterosexual sex games involving some kind of female domination, if only from time to time. That this to some extent reflects the rise in women's assertiveness generally in society cannot be doubted, but whatever the reasons, and they are many, there is currently considerable interest in the subject.

In the USA there are about 100 specialist magazines catering for this taste, each with a circulation of about 10,000 to 20,000, and one researcher who looked at this aspect of sexuality in detail over many years suggests that about 100,000 to 150,000 males visit professional dominant women or mistresses for erotic satisfaction in any one year. Just how such figures translate to other countries is not known.

About two-thirds of all the fantasies reported by Nancy Friday in her book *Men in Love: Their Secret Fantasies* (Quartet 1976) contained elements of male submission. To be fair, this is hardly a statistically valid sample of males, and studies of whole populations do not back up this sort of proportion. A 1976 *Playboy* study of college students found that 1 in 12 of the young women asked said they had fantasies on inflicting pain on men. Once again one should not extrapolate this figure to apply to all women of all ages and educational levels.

The vast majority of men who enjoy this sort of submissive sexual role, in reality or in fantasy, are normal heterosexuals in a one-to-one relationship. They combine their sexual submissiveness with their traditional male-dominant role. The problem is that very, very few partners of such men want to indulge their fantasy, either in reverie or in real life. It appears that most females find the whole subject abhorrent.

Just why such men enjoy being submissive isn't completely understood. For some it is a release from their day-to-day responsibilities and restrictions; others find submission a way of compensating for their usual aggressive, dominant or manipulative behaviour; others have an unconscious need to be punished; some see their punishment as atonement for their feelings of guilt at having hurt others, and so on. However, for many men I think it's the letting go, the lying back and allowing someone else to be in charge while they abandon themselves to their feelings, that's so exciting. Indeed, some such men say their very best orgasms come from these sorts of experiences, and a few talk of transcendental experiences never attainable in any other form of sexual encounter.

Abe's fantasy reflects his real experiences with his mistress, whom he visits several times a year for punishment:

STERN MISTRESS

My fantasy involves my mistress, who's a real expert. She knows exactly what I like and takes every detail seriously. She strips me naked and carefully puts a collar round my neck, talking to me all the time about how she's going to punish me. Just hearing her talk about it makes me have an erection, but if I look like getting too excited too soon she applies a special harness to my prick and balls, which restrains my erection.

When she's applied all the restraining straps, she starts on her tantalizingly slow torture that increases my arousal. First she applies a clip to each nipple, and then starts to strap me with her favourite leather thong. As I become more aroused, the amount of pain I can take increases and the very nature of it changes. I go into a spaced-out state, in which the pain becomes pleasure.

Now she makes me bend down in front of her and kiss her thigh-high boots. As I kneel before her she shouts at me if I don't kiss her feet and legs properly, and threatens further punishment as she makes me get the kisses just perfect, right up to her bare thighs. As I presume to approach too close to her crotch she gives me a sharp crack on the behind with her whip to bring me back into control.

'You know you aren't allowed there,' she chides me. 'You'll regret you did that, you little worm.' With this she bends me over to touch my toes and starts to play with my anus. 'I thought I told you to shave your balls last time you were here,' she barks, as she inserts two fingers into my rectum and starts to stimulate my prostate gland.

Seeing my erection is now enormous she swings her cane across my balls as they hang down between my legs. I scream out in agony, because they're aroused and tender as hell.

'I'll give you something to yell about, you wimp,' she taunts, and so saying thrusts a giant dildo into my anus and works it in and out. I nearly pass out with the sensations and at this stage usually come.

WHIPPING AND SPANKING

These types of fantasy are quite complicated. It is certainly true that some people unconsciously link love and punishment (*see* page 84), but there are probably other mechanisms at work, too. For the individual on the receiving end, the pain can smother any anxiety or guilt they feel about their sexual arousal, but I think physiological mechanisms might also play a part.

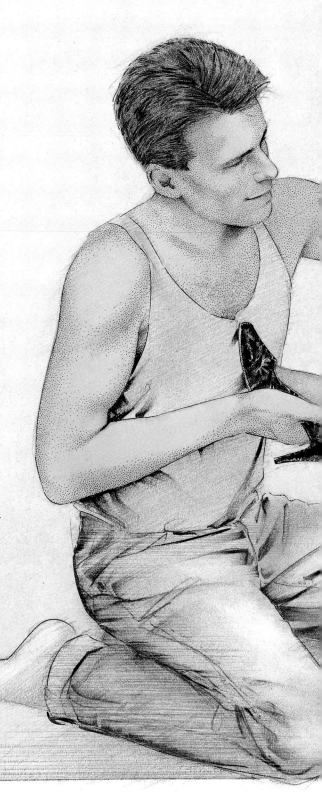

She is playing the stern mistress making him undress her slowly and teasingly, exactly as she directs. If he does it really well she will reward him with sex.

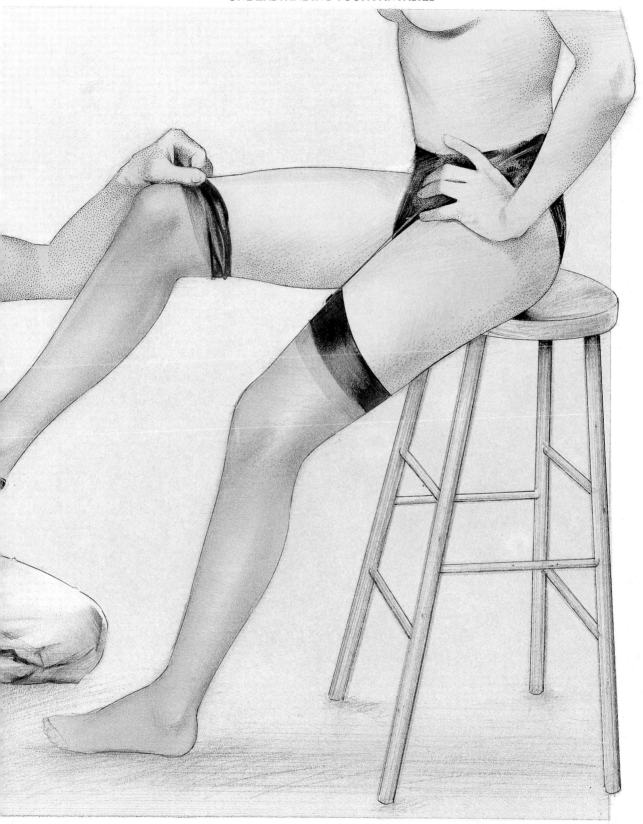

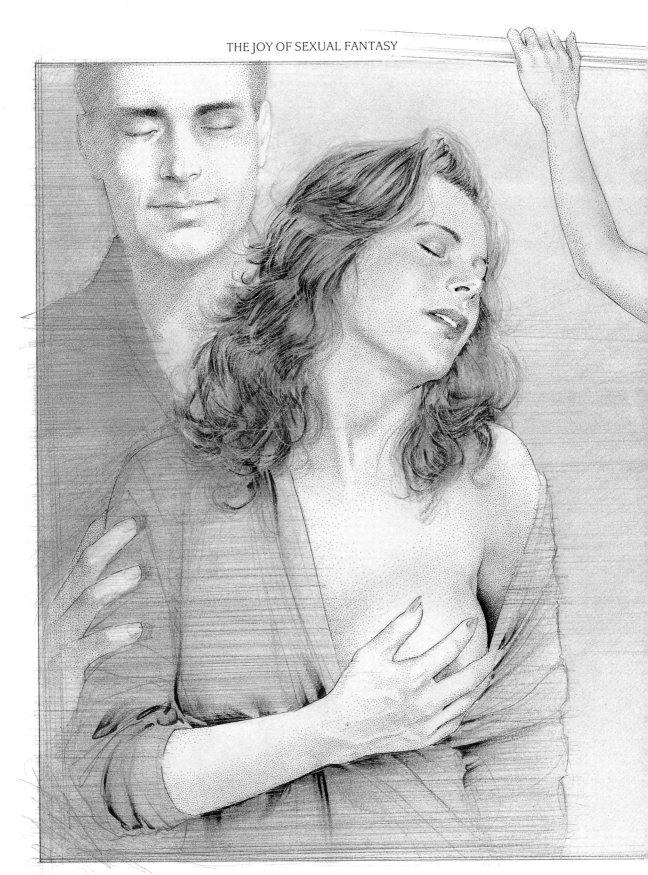

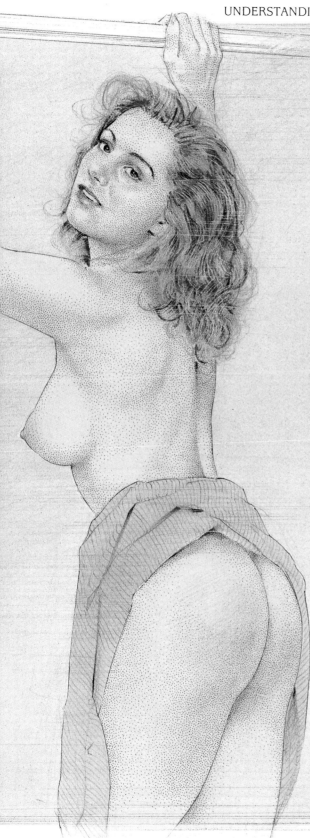

During sexual arousal, the pelvic organs swell and fill with blood. Therefore, this blood-filled state becomes associated with sexual excitement. Smacked buttocks also become red with hot blood. It's hardly very fanciful to suggest that this becomes confused in the brain with sexual arousal. Being smacked or whipped causes stress hormone levels in the blood to rise. These increase sex hormone production, which causes a feeling of arousal.

Aggression is an integral part of mammalian sex. The males of certain species inflict bites or other types of pain on their females when copulating. Indeed, aggression has been found, in several laboratory experiments, to be highly arousing in humans. Psychologists have carried out experiments to investigate the relationship between aggression and arousal: first questioning a group of people to find out how aroused they feel, then stressing them by subjecting them to someone acting aggressively towards them; and requestioning them about how aroused they then feel. The conclusion is that aggression enhances arousal considerably.

Ritualizing this primitive aggression, in fact or fantasy, is therefore to be expected as a part of normal sexual relationships. The increased blood flow to the genital area produced by spanking or whipping can be added to more deep-rooted unconscious material from our mammalian heritage, and from infancy and childhood, to make such fantasies valuable.

WHIPPED UP TO PASSION

My fantasy is based on a video I saw once at my friend's house. It's about a girl of about 19 called Judy, who was very naughty at her sex classes. She had this very strict male teacher, Art, who tested her on her sexual homework. If she hadn't done it properly he would punish her severely.

One day she hadn't completed her required reading of *The Story of O*, though in my fantasy I think she did it deliberately so that she would be punished. In the video the girl

Spanking is a common love game, but for some, the fantasy takes things just that bit further to enhance the value of the reverie.

certainly wanted to be punished for being so naughty. When Art can no longer bear to hear Judy's pathetic excuses about why she hasn't done her homework, he tells her that she will have to be taken down to his dungeon, where she will be dealt with in a way that will remind her to do her work properly in future. She looks rather scared at the prospect, but deep down I know she wants it.

The next scene is in the dungeon. It's dark and there are lots of different sex gadgets and toys around the place. First, Art makes her change into some sexy black underwear and high-heeled black shoes. She comes back from the dressing-room with both her breasts out of the bra, so Art can see them easily, but he gets furious with her because the seams of her stockings aren't straight.

'Put your stockings on properly,' he orders, flicking her ass sharply with a riding crop.

As she bends down to do this he cracks the crop across her right breast. She winces with the pain. When she stands up again she looks a lot neater, and Art inspects her minutely.

'Turn around slowly so I can look at you properly,' he commands.

She does as she's told.

'To the cross,' he bids, motioning to a large, wooden, x-shaped structure against the wall.

She walks to it and when she's there he inserts a gag into her mouth. When it is tied securely behind her head he tells her to turn around.

'Let's test it out and see what we can hear. I don't want to hear any of your pathetic crying.' So saying, he brings the riding crop down on her left breast, this time much harder than before. She screams in agony. 'It needs tightening,' he says, and does it up one more notch on the leather strap at the back of her head. 'Now go to the cross and face me.'

He now ties her up so that her hands are reaching as far up as they will go, stretched tightly against the black, heavy wooden cross. 'Open your legs,' he commands, and when she has done so he ties them to the lower limbs of the wooden structure. Judy is now spread-eagled against the cross, dressed only in her bra, pulled down to reveal her breasts, and her garter belt, stockings and high-heeled shoes.

'Now for your punishment. You'll never forget to do your homework after this, I can assure you,' he sneers.

Judy begins to shake with fear and excite-ment. She knows that she's asked for this and wants it to be done, but is still afraid of what he'll do.

Art now selects a long, thin cane from his collection and stands at one side of her. He plays with her nipple on that side, teasing it gently with the cane and making it erect. 'You like your body whipped and beaten, don't you, Judy?' he asks.

'Yes, master,' she replies, muffled with the tight gag.

'What did you say?' he shouts.

'Yes, master,' she replies as loudly as she can with the gag in place.

'Yes you do. You love being tied up and beaten. It makes you want to come, doesn't it now?'

'Yes, master,' she mouths more quietly under the supple leather gag, nodding her head at the same time.

'Then we mustn't disappoint you, must we?' he says, stopping the cane from caressing her nipple for a second.

Just as Judy thinks he's stopped arousing her in the cruel and sadistic way she so enjoys, she feels the sharp edge of the bamboo bite into her nipple as he canes it viciously. She yells with pain. He crosses to her other side and starts playing with the other nipple in the same way as before.

'We can't ignore this one, can we?' he torments her. 'We don't want this one to be jealous,' and with a cruel swish of the cane sends her body writhing in anguish as her other nipple shudders under the blow.

Judy is now gently sobbing and obviously doesn't want any more. He stops for a moment and starts to caress her breasts and nipples with his hands.

'That better?' he asks, as he takes her sore nipples one in each hand and rolls them between finger and thumb, pulling them until she squirms with the pain.

'I expect your little pussy is ready to come now, Judy,' he says, feeling her vagina with several fingers. She is wet and highly excited. She wriggles with delight as he delves into her gaping hole. 'You don't think you're going to come like this?' he taunts. 'No you're not.'

Now he has a riding crop in his hand and starts to deliver soft blows all over her belly, breasts and inner thighs. Slowly her whole body reddens with the repeated strokes of the crop. She arches her back and her breathing quickens. He pays more attention to her inner thighs and, working his way up her crotch, starts expertly to whip her vulva from right between her legs at the back, forwards to her clitoris.

She shakes and trembles with pleasure as he rains blow after expert blow on her genitals, until she climaxes with a crying moan.

He continues to pay her genitals the attention they so crave, not stopping with the crop until her body comes to rest, exhausted from her orgasms.

Louisa's fantasy demonstrates how pleasure and pain are inextricably linked in the minds of some individuals. She is, in real life, very unsure of her right to enjoy sex. She was taught as a child that sex is bad and she avoids it whenever possible. She masturbates hardly at all and can't maintain a sexual relationship for any length of time. For her, as for many women with this kind of unconscious belief structure, if she is to enjoy sex and become aroused she must be punished for it. Some such women have been smacked or punished in other ways by their parents or other authority figures, for their interest in sex, but this is not always the case.

MY IDEAL PUNISHMENT

I've been a naughty girl and my ex-lover is really cross with me. He tells me that I have to fellate him but, try as I will, I can't do it to his liking. This means that I must be punished. In fact I didn't do it properly in the first place because I really wanted the punishment. I know that afterwards I'll fellate him in the way he likes, but the punishment must come first.

'Come over here,' he commands in a stern voice. Then, 'Go and lie over there, face down on that stool.'

I cross to a double piano stool and lie on it.

'Spread your legs,' he barks.

I do so, letting them fall to either side of the stool.

'Now I'll show you what happens to naughty girls who don't know how to suck me,' he teases. And coming up to my exposed behind, he slaps it quite hard with the flat of his hand. It isn't too bad, but it stings a bit. 'How was that?' he demands.

'Quite painful,' I reply.

'That's only the beginning. You just wait till I start to make it really red and warm.'

He then begins to spank me really hard. The blows come one after the other until I think I can take no more. I start to get up so as to escape the pain.

'If you move one inch I'll tie you down,' he threatens. And I know he will, so I stay put. After a while he stops smacking me. 'How's your little cunt? Is it wet yet?' he teases. He then puts a couple of fingers into me and feels every inch of my cunt. The juices flow out of it and I know this is why I like the spanking.

'You'll soon be ready to suck me properly, won't you?' he whispers in my ear.

'Yes,' I moan, as he gives me one last smack on my red, sore behind.

Now he lies on his back on the floor and orders me to kneel over him with my fanny facing his head. 'Suck me properly now or you'll get more of the same treatment.'

I do what he says and suck him beautifully. As I am busy at this arousing task he tells me that it's not good enough, and before I know it he's smacking my behind again. The pain now is much worse than before and I want it to stop. I know that the only way he'll stop is if I make him come in my mouth, so I work expertly at his prick to excite him quickly. As he comes in my mouth he gives me one last smack and I have my own orgasm.

TERROR AND FRIGHT

These themes constitute another area that is closely associated with SM fantasies. They link the notions of death and sex, a powerful combination that cannot be denied. Horror movies and stories play on the connection. The whole subject is covered in more detail on page 35.

Fear and terror are perhaps very elegant, unconscious ways in which people can yield to sexual forces they couldn't otherwise face. After all, who could blame anyone for having to undertake sexual acts if the alternative is to die? I find that such fantasies are rare outside highly inhibited individuals or perhaps those with a high sense of melodrama. The two characteristics can go together, especially in women.

RAVISHED BY FEAR

I don't know how this fantasy came about in the first place, but I must say that I get turned on by scary things generally. I love it on a roller coaster, or at horror movies, for example, and I'm often aroused when other people are scared by something.

Still, whatever the explanation, my fantasy is about this man breaking into my house one night. I wake up to find him going through the drawers in my room. I'm terrified. What should I do? Scream for the neighbours? Keep quiet and let him get away with it? Try to get to the bedside phone to call the police?

The intruder goes about his business and then, to my horror, comes over to the bedside table to look for valuables. I nearly die trying to keep quiet as he approaches the bed. I try desperately to breathe normally, but I can't, I'm beside myself with fear. Although my eyes are closed he must sense that I'm not asleep, because with one movement he whisks the bedclothes off my naked body, leaving me totally helpless.

'Keep your eyes closed, or you'll never see again,' he growls menacingly. He then ties a blindfold over my eyes and starts to handle my body.

I writhe around trying to avoid his filthy, exploring hands. This makes him furious. 'You'd better not give me any trouble or I'll cut you to pieces, you little slut.'

With this I feel the cold steel of a large knife on my throat. He draws it across my skin very gently to show me what it is he's talking about. 'One move and you're a goner,' he says.

The next thing I know, my legs are being forced apart and something is being put inside me. It isn't his penis. I don't know what it is but it's large and it hurts. I struggle some more and start to cry out, but stop abruptly when I feel the cold blade on my left breast.

'Any more silly business and I'll cut your tits off.'

I'm now so afraid that I start sobbing uncontrollably. Weak with fear and drained of energy, I'm quite powerless to do anything. He sees that I've finally given in and gets between my legs and has sex with me.

To my eternal shame and guilt I'm aroused as hell and he notices it.

'You love all this, don't you, you little whore?' he says, toying with my breasts once more with his knife. My nipples ache unbearably as the cold metal touches them. They're already erect as the blade swishes over them, but they try to get even bigger.

The combination of his prick in me and the sheer terror of him actually cutting my breasts makes me climax in a way I never normally do. When I masturbate I sometimes use this fantasy and stroke my breast and nipple with an ordinary blunt table knife or some other object while I come.

UNDRESSING

Many childhood games involve putting on and taking off clothes. Doctors and nurses, dressing-up games, 'I'll show you mine if you'll show me yours', are all popular children's games today and probably always have been. Adults, however, keep their bodies clothed, not just to keep out the cold or to adorn themselves, but to exclude others from a knowledge of their sexual anatomy. Even in cultures in which only a loincloth is worn, people jealously guard their genital privacy; it's considered the height of bad manners to do anything else.

Fantasies that involve undressing or being undressed are found fairly commonly in both sexes. The victim loves it in the fantasy, even if in real life the situation would be unbearably embarrassing. To a large extent, such fantasies embody at least some degree of sadism or masochism, yet by all accounts this element is usually not very gross.

Whether or not people who have these fantasies experienced having been undressed seductively in childhood is often hard to discover. Certainly, some have memories of such experiences, but I suspect the majority have not. Perhaps the link is between parental love/sex in the Oedipal stage of psychosexual development (*see* page 41) and a learned response to the business of dressing or of being undressed by a parent of the opposite sex. This link enables the fantasist to deal with unresolved issues surrounding this childhood period. For the individual who felt loved, cherished and perhaps even aroused while being dressed and undressed by a parent, this fantasy could serve to deal with such forbidden ideas under a relatively acceptable guise.

The re-creation of a forbidden behaviour can reverberate back to childhood and help combat old anxieties or live out old dreams. It's my impression that those who have had a liberal upbringing, with parental nudity as a normal, accepted part of family life, don't find much pleasure in undressing or being undressed in their fantasies. Concepts of naughtiness and anxiety associated with dressing and undressing are much lower in children from a liberal background, so the subject is far less taboo and thus less exciting as a fantasy.

A few people make their undressing fantasy an integral part of their daily lives. Glamour models and strippers, for example, earn a living acting out such fantasies. Terri wasn't a model, but very much wanted to be one:

THE PRIZE SPECIMEN

In this fantasy, and it's just one of many I have, I'm a top model going for a job at an advertising agency. I'm gorgeous and irresistible and take with me photos of other jobs I've done for various clients.

I get to the agency and am shown into an office, where there are several men and one woman sitting around a sort of conference table.

'Come in and sit down, Terri,' one of the men says.

'Could we see some of your work first?' another one asks.

I open the portfolio and display my best ads, one of me in stockings for a well known firm; in underwear for a catalogue; and in a bikini for a swimwear company. They pass the photos around and admire them.

'I think we should see for ourselves what she's really like,' the young man says.

'Exactly,' says another and turns to the woman. 'Jill, would you take Terri over there and undress her slowly so we can see what will look best for the ad?'

Jill comes over to me and leads me to the centre of the room. The lights dim as if by magic; one spotlight is trained on the two of us. Jill is attractive and very ad-agency svelte, definitely college educated and has model-quality looks. She starts to unbutton my jacket and parts it to expose my blouse.

'That's good,' says one of the men. 'Now ease it off her shoulders.'

Jill does as she's told and the group admires my figure. I never wear a bra, so my breasts show up well under the blouse and I can't help noticing my nipples are slightly erect.

'The blouse next, Jill,' the boss orders.

She slowly and seductively undoes the buttons and, going behind me, eases the fabric off my shoulders so that my breasts peep out teasingly.

'That would be a great shot,' one of the men suggests.

'Too obvious,' says another. 'Let's try something more subtle than that.'

Jill now removes my blouse completely and starts to undo the waistband of my skirt. As she slips it off, the men murmur appreciatively as it reveals my black lacy panties and stockings. I must admit that I have stunning thighs and legs, which is why I get all the stocking ads.

'That's better,' says one guy, who is obviously the photographer, judging by his comments about technicalities. 'Take her panties off now.'

Jill reaches down to pull them off me and just as she does this, the photographer yells, 'Stop! That's the shot – with her panties just pulled down to reveal a bit of pubic hair and her legs slightly open. Part your legs for us, honey. Just a bit. That's perfect.'

I do so and suddenly realize that, although I'm a professional model, this is really turning me on. At this point I usually climax, but if I let it run any more it usually includes one of the men taking me over to the table and removing my panties as I lie facing everyone, to reveal my pussy to their delighted gaze.

SAME-SEX ACTIVITIES

I don't call these 'homosexual' fantasies, because, in the commonly accepted sense of the word, 'homosexual' means so much more than simply having fantasies about, or sex with, someone of the same sex. Being homosexual usually means adopting a particular kind of lifestyle and mixing with a subculture of like-minded people. Simply having same-sex fantasies doesn't mean that the heterosexual fantasist is destined to become a part of this subculture or give up the heterosexual life.

It can hardly be disputed by most thinking people that everyone is capable of a range of sexual activities with people of either sex. Most young boys in their early teens go through a period of same-sex experimentation as they learn about their sexuality: counting pubic hairs; indulging in 'how far can you pee' games; comparing penis size; and much more, short of sexual intercourse. Girls don't experience quite the same process, but in late teens and early adulthood same-sex activities at colleges and other residential establishments are so common as to be thought normal.

In both cases the overwhelming majority of individuals who experiment in this way end up exclusively heterosexual in their practical genital orientation. What their unconscious has in store may be quite another matter, however, and it's the unconscious that surfaces in fantasy.

Whether everyone has fantasies of this nature or not, all individuals are capable of exhibiting the same-sex side of their sexual nature at almost any time. In Western culture this is much more acceptable among females who are allowed to cuddle, kiss, walk arm in arm, caress and indulge in other expressions of emotional intimacy without much criticism. Similar behaviour in males is largely forbidden, and this shuts many men out of emotionally rewarding relationships. This is a disservice to males almost everywhere in the West.

So, on a scale which starts at 'all same-sex activities and fantasies' and progresses through to 'only heterosexual activities and fantasies', each person finds his or her unique place. And this changes from time to time and age to age. For those who lie somewhere near the homosexual end of the scale, yet live a mainly heterosexual life, perhaps being married with a family, fantasies involving individuals of the same sex enable them to cope both with what they have and with their unconscious needs.

In a largely heterosexual culture, same-sex fantasies arouse considerable anxiety, suspicion, fear and guilt. They are, as a result, suppressed or find expression indirectly.

I see many women who, after discovering what they think is a lesbian fantasy, become alarmed and ask me if they're about to change their sexual orientation. That the fantasy is so powerful, and gives them rewards that their heterosexual fantasies and real-life experiences do not, only adds fuel to an already dangerous-feeling fire.

Reassurance usually works wonders. In fact I give such women books to read about real lesbian life. Almost without exception they are deeply moved by what they read and come quickly to regard their same-sex fantasies as a very loving, real and acceptable part of being a sexual female. This experience also seems to bring them in touch, often for the first time, with other women and their sexuality, something they had never been able to do because, in my view, it was too dangerous even to think about other women in this way.

Most women who have same-sex fantasies do little or nothing about them in real life. They don't seek the sexual company of other women at all. Quite the contrary – they use such fantasies to enhance their heterosexual life with their partner.

Men, on the other hand, are much more likely to want to do something about their new-found toy. This is partly because men tend to be sexual initiators anyway, and partly because there are enough men around who will take part in genitally based, same-sex activities. I don't suggest that all men who have same-sex fantasies are bound to act them out. This isn't so. Many young men have at least some same-sex fantasies and wonder if they're going to become gay, but of course they aren't. Sometimes these fantasies arise because when a young man's sexual potency is at its peak in his late teens and early twenties, he may not have sufficient opportunity or social skills to create sexual outlets with women. Bad experiences with young and inexperienced women can put him off females; so can old, unconscious material from dealing with his own, mother or other significant women. He can also find himself going off women, if only for a while, because they're 'too much trouble'. At this stage of life same-sex fantasies become an attractive alternative.

Barbara's fantasy is fairly typical for a girl in her late teens, keen on her best friend, who is also her flatmate:

A FRIEND IN NEED

I'm not a lesbian, but from time to time I fantasize about making love with my best friend. We're very close in real life but we have never done anything sexual with each other.

In my fantasy I'm in bed with her one sunny afternoon. She's kissing my shoulders and all down my back as I lie on my stomach. She runs her fingers down my spine and caresses the base of my back with small, firm, circular movements on either side of the spine. It's bliss and I feel myself becoming aroused.

As I lie there revelling in it all, her hand slips between my thighs, which I part slightly to welcome her exploring fingers. Feeling my juices run warm and moist out of my vagina, she asks me to turn on to my back. I'm in ecstasy as she runs her tongue all over my breasts and nipples, teasing its way around my tummy button and down towards my pubic area, without actually touching it. The insides of my thighs are the next to receive her attention. She licks the insides of the backs of my knees. This nearly drives me wild; I can hardly bear it any longer.

Now her body is parting my legs as she edges up towards my cunt. In seconds her tongue is on my lips, stroking them and licking my clitoris with long, wet movements. I feel her moist mouth close to my own wetness and love the thought of our wetness mingling. I hold her tightly as my orgasm approaches and as I shake with ecstasy I push her face more and more into my vagina, so that she can feel me coming.

WATCHING AND BEING WATCHED

The origins of voyeurism are complex and largely unknown. The forbidden nature of sex in Western culture doesn't help the study of voyeurism, but why it is that watching others having sex is so fascinating is something of a mystery. It's certainly more than the fact that sex is private and that most people are nosey.

Very few people find it easy to avert their gaze from a couple engaged in sexual activity. It is, after all, a largely hidden matter, scarcely seen in public. In the days when families all lived and slept together, no doubt voyeuristic fantasies were rare, but today the mystery is powerful and makes the sexual activities of others fascinating fantasy material.

Adult movies and videos play on this in a very obvious way: many a love story with sex scenes becomes a substitute, in my view, for what most people would have witnessed in the family bedroom a few hundred years ago.

The thrill of the forbidden undoubtedly plays its part, but it's not just that we obtain vicarious pleasure from seeing others have pleasure. Many people like to watch to com-pare themselves and their sexual functioning with that of others; there's a lot to be learned from observation.

For some people watching is preferable to doing, and not just in the sexual arena. Watching an exciting motor race on TV, or, better still, at the race circuit, is a good substitute for risking one's own neck by cornering at 140 miles an hour. It's much the same with spectator sex. And people who are concerned with their sexual competence or performance can more easily feel at ease watching other people put themselves on the line than if they were expected to do so themselves.

In fact, given that sex is such a complex activity, it's really quite extraordinary that society allows people almost no opportunity to witness it firsthand, as a way of learning about it. What people can't learn about they tend to worry about. In 'watching' fantasies the dreamer tries to defuse this anxiety.

Of course, the person or people whom fantasists are watching are also essential to an understanding of these fantasies. I find that the people an individual chooses to eavesdrop on in their voyeuristic fantasies yield helpful information when interpreting the fantasy.

Watching others having fantasy sex is not simply a matter of looking in on any non-specific couple's love-making, it has much more to do with looking in on one's own innermost personality. In an unconscious psychological sense, it's possible to 'make love to yourself' in such scenarios. Under such a guise individuals can cope with the masculine and feminine parts of their personality in a way that's almost impossible otherwise.

It's often said that women are basically exhibitionistic and men largely voyeuristic, but this is far too simple a stereotype. Certainly, women in Western culture are encouraged – often by men – to show off their bodies, and dress in male-created fashions. But the catch is that they're supposed to do it without appearing pushy or unduly seductive. It's also a fact that men like to exhibit their women as a way of displaying their own sexual prowess. This has the effect of reflecting attention from the woman on to her man. In this way, women are trophies for such men. A common fantasy for men is seeing themselves with a very beautiful woman, probably one far more attractive than they would be able to obtain in real life.

To some extent everyone is a voyeur. Men

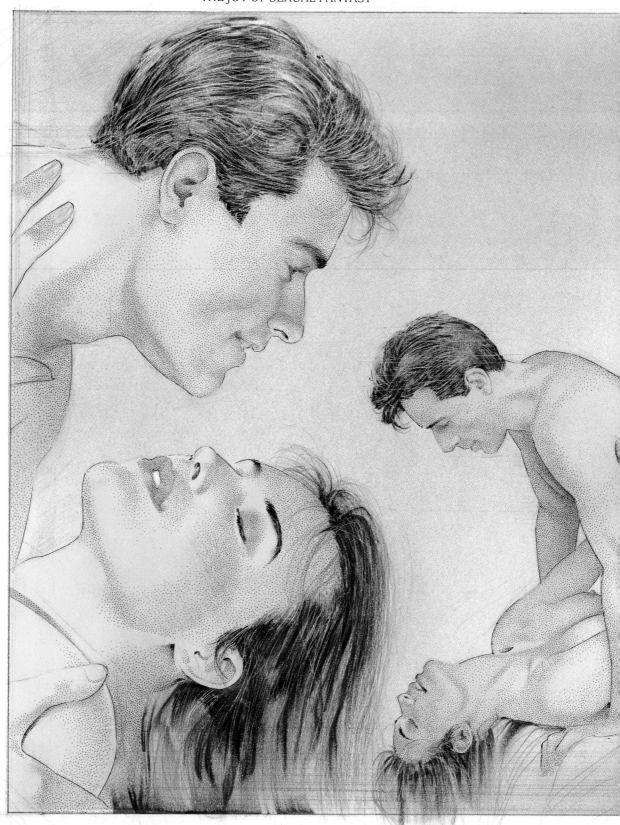

and women look at attractive people of the same and the opposite sex. Indeed, there are few more attentive watchers of women than other women. For a large minority of men, voyeurism is an almost daily part of their lives. Girlie magazines present females to male gaze and masturbation fantasy. In fact, such women are probably the largest single external source of male masturbation fantasies.

Many women have fantasies of being admired and found sexually attractive by men, and sometimes by many men at once. Stripper fantasies are not uncommon, and many of my female patients have told me that they fantasize about being so attractive and sexy that men cannot resist them.

Real-life women can, of course, reject men who seek their sexual favours. In a voyeuristic fantasy there's no such danger. The man has all the power and needn't fear being put down, failing sexually, or being rejected. This is one of the reasons that girlie magazines have such a perennial appeal. In a similar way females are emotional voyeurs when reading romantic fiction.

Watching and being watched will always be popular fantasies for both sexes. Changes in women's sexual roles in and out of the bedroom mean that they take a much more frank and open interest in male bodies than was previously apparent. In my work in various spheres, not just in my practice, I now find that women are much more aggressive voyeuristically than even ten years ago. Tales of hen nights recounted to me by male strippers certainly leave little to the imagination and prove, if proof were needed, that women are, and always have been, just as interested in looking as in showing. Today, perhaps for the first time in history, they have the opportunity to be open about it.

Anna's story is really her husband's fantasy, but she finds herself involved in it when they have sex:

A SEXY SAMPLE

My husband's favourite fantasy, which he asks me to talk him through when we're having sex, is all about me being a subject in a sex laboratory.

The fantasy starts off as he takes me to this sex lab where people are carrying out experiments on female sexual response. I leave him in a sound-proof observation room just outside the lab so he can see what happens, but a one-way mirror prevents me from seeing him.

The doctor running the test comes in and

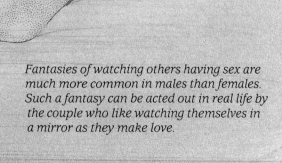

Fantasies of watching others having sex are much more common in males than females. Such a fantasy can be acted out in real life by the couple who like watching themselves in a mirror as they make love.

asks me to take my clothes off. I do this eagerly because I'm excited about what is to happen. He then asks me to lie on a large bed or couch and attaches all kinds of wires to me and inserts a sensor into my vagina.

As I recount this part of the story I tell my husband exactly how it feels having my nipples attached to the electrical leads and what the probe feels like as it goes inside me.

The doctor turns me toward the two-way mirror, so that my husband can clearly see everything that's going on.

Now comes the experiment. A highly attractive young man in his early twenties comes in. He undresses in a very matter-of-fact way and displays his half-erect penis. The doctor asks me to make him erect and I offer to do this by fellating him. The man guides me down on to my knees in front of him so my face is level with his penis. I then suck him until he's big.

When his erection is large enough the doctor tells us to get on to the bed and start having sex. He then leaves the room and we get down to business.

At this point in the story I describe all kinds of sexual goings on between me and this young buck as he fucks me every which way.

At some stage during all of this my husband ejaculates. He tells me that this fantasy gives him the biggest turn-on.

PHYSICAL MATERIALS AND CLOTHING

The fascination of physical materials and clothing as fetish objects in real life or in fantasy is a source of bewilderment to most people. At first, the notion that anyone could become sexually aroused at the thought of a shoe, a nappy, a rubber sheet or a silk blouse seems preposterous. So where do these seemingly extraordinary tastes originate?

There are several theories, but in my opinion it's largely a learned phenomenon, usually acquired very early in life. This is why such fantasies are so resistant to change – they are embedded deep in the unconscious.

For some men – I say 'men' because fetishistic fantasies are vastly more popular with men than with women – the fantasy object is simply an addition to their normal

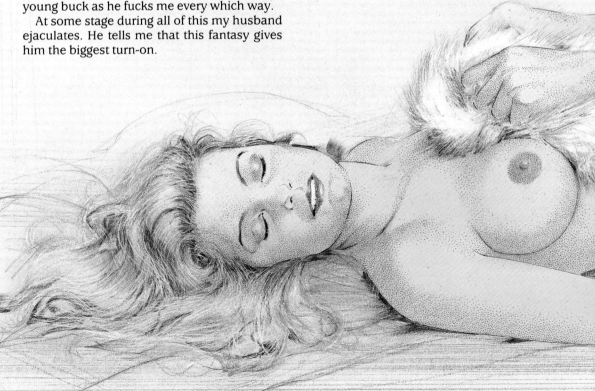

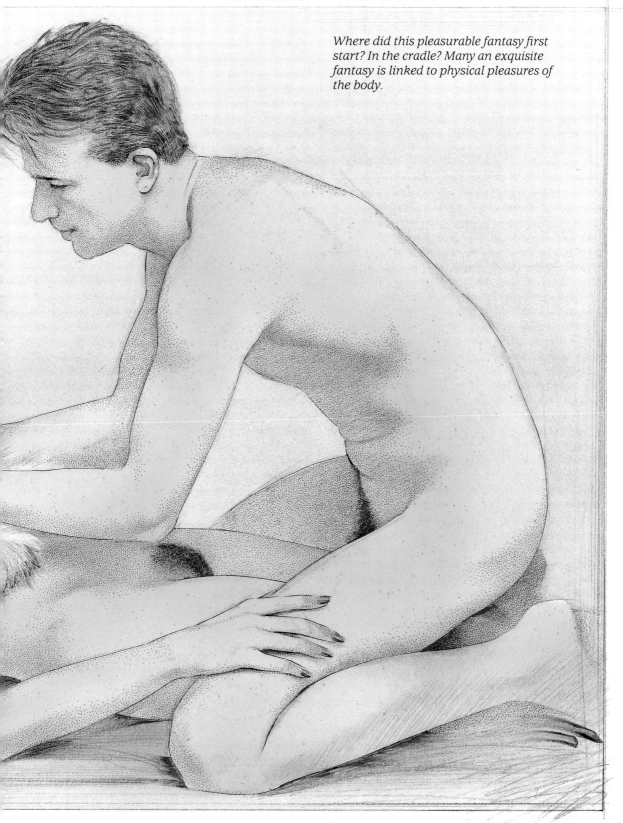

Where did this pleasurable fantasy first start? In the cradle? Many an exquisite fantasy is linked to physical pleasures of the body.

sexual menu, a sort of enhancer. There's clearly little problem with this, whether it occurs in fact or fantasy. After all, enhancers are used by most people, if only from time to time, to spice up their sexual and romantic lives. However, to the true fetishist, the fantasy object is a fixed necessity, without which he cannot function or, if he can, is unable to obtain pleasure. The true fetishist isn't turned on by a shoe because it's worn by his lady, but because of its 'shoeness'.

Just what the fetish object represents in the unconscious of a man with this sort of fantasy is anyone's guess. Some claim that such sex is 'safe' for the man because it doesn't involve him in sexual activity with a real woman. Whether such concerns about and fears of women originate in unconscious castration anxiety, as some psychoanalysts assert, is impossible to say.

I cannot deny that there might be some truth in this theory, but my clinical work shows me that learned experiences and events are far more likely to hold the key. Many such men have real-life experiences of fearing the loss of their mother, rather than of their penis, in my view. I get back to this using regression techniques in hypnosis. The fetish object then comes to represent a symbolic comforter that takes the place of the mother who wasn't a real comfort in earliest infancy and childhood. Just as a little child who is insecure hangs on to a security blanket or 'cuddly', so the adult fetishist clings to his object, reinforcing its value by linking it with sex.

Of all the items chosen as fetish objects, the most common is a woman's shoe. It's not known why this is, but it might be that from an infant's point of view it's the part of his mother he sees most. This is particularly likely to be true of the rejecting, non-intimate mother, in whose arms and at whose breast he spends so little time.

Similarly, it's possible that women's underwear could come to be associated with fetishistic pleasure in an 'as if it were my mother' way in a male. Whether this dates from a baby boy's earliest experiences of the physical texture of her underwear, or his later Oedipal memories of her walking around clad only in underwear during a period when he's making sexual connections with her in his mind, is open to debate.

However it comes about, certain male babies and young boys learn to re-create the closeness, warmth and even perhaps the smells of their mother's body as they snuggle up to their fetish object. It's as if some ancient part of the brain is triggered, rather as in a bird returning to the same nest each year.

To me, the most interesting part of all this is why there are so few female fetishists. As women behave more like men in society there's undoubtedly an increase in women's reports of fetishism, but they're still only a tiny fraction of those reported by men. It could be that female children are permitted to make sensuous, even sexual contact with such materials as a part of growing up, and so don't have the craving for them in adult life. I have no reason to believe that girl babies are any less vulnerable to separation from or rejection by their mothers, but it could be that they cope with it better. After all, boys go through a stage of falling in love with mother as an extension of having been in love with her for different reasons since birth. Girl babies, in contrast, lose their mothers when they 'fall in love with Daddy' at the Oedipal stage of their psychosexual development. From then on females are essentially rivals for the rest of their lives, whereas many boys and, indeed, men, continue to be in love with their mothers all their lives.

A facet of fetishistic fantasy that makes me think it is mainly a learned phenomenon is the quite extraordinary detail that such men invest in their object, and the surroundings in which it is sexually attractive. If, as has been suggested, the object represents the mother in some sort of symbolic way, it's perhaps not too surprising that the individual invests it with loving detail. In a sense, he's describing his ideal mother when fantasizing in this way about his fetish object. If you love someone, the details of their clothing, perfume, movements, hairstyle and other idiosyncrasies become very important.

Society favours all this quite unconsciously. The importance of shoes and feet is quite extraordinary when looked at throughout history, let alone today. The ancient Chinese, for example, bound the feet of their females so that they couldn't walk. The sexual significance of this was paramount. Men used to compare the bound, doubled-over foot with the vulva, and there are records of the delights of sexual intercourse with such feet. In today's world the sight of a high-heeled shoe can arouse many men, whether or not it contains the foot of a woman they desire. Many women, especially, tell me how erotic their feet are when caressed, and I know several who have orgasmic or near-orgasmic experiences from foot massage.

The subject of fetishes, then, is a fascinating one. It will continue to baffle us, no doubt, and because of this its strange, inexplicable magic will always be a fantasy favourite.

For an example of how a material experienced in childhood can create adult fantasies and fetishes *see* page 16.

INCEST

In Western culture today there are really only two remaining taboos: death and incest. Almost every other area has been exposed to public gaze and accepted in one form or another. Sex with a prohibited member of a family still arouses strong feelings, yet the subject figures in a fantasy most people have had at one time or another.

It's almost univeral for children aged between three and five to wish they could possess their opposite-sex parent, while banishing their same-sex one. This appears to be a crucial stage in growing up. What most people don't realize is that the very essence of this Oedipal love is that it must never be actualized. To do so is to condemn the individual to a lifetime of sexual tyranny as a result of having won the battle against the same-sex parent. Such individuals go through life believing that they can split up any other love-bonded couple. After all, if as a little girl you can win out over your own mother, whose relationship is ever safe?

It's at this stage of their development that children learn, or should learn, about love triangles: that some people are unobtainable. It is the psychological frustration of not being able to possess their opposite-sex parent that leads people to look elsewhere – outside the family – for another partner.

Unfortunately, this process is ruined for many girls because their fathers, or other significant adult males, teach them to use their sexuality to destroy adult relationships. What was and should have remained a fantasy becomes a reality and, in my clinical experience, cripples many such women in the sense that they're unable ever to distinguish between the two again.

While everyone has fantasies of some sort about an opposite-sex parent, in early childhood or later in adolescence, most people consciously banish such material because it's so socially unacceptable. Whenever I hear someone claim that they don't fantasize I suspect I'm not far away from an incest fantasy. It's also interesting to note that whenever people are asked in questionnaires about their fantasies they hardly ever volunteer incest as a theme. I have never come across a study in which incest figures with any prominence.

In therapy it rarely takes long to uncover the hidden symbolism of forbidden sex objects. The readiness with which patients enter into parental sex fantasy relationships with the therapist is one example of how this makes itself known. In families in which a child, especially a girl, is exposed to her father's sexuality in a very obvious way – for example, if she slept in the same room as her parents much past babyhood – these incest fantasies are never far away.

Some mothers are too intrusive into their little boys' sexuality. For example, they make personal enquiries about their masturbation habits and thoughts, under the guise of loving interest. Such a boy can easily become over-involved with his mother and have incestuous fantasies about her.

In many families today the father is largely absent. As a result some young boys grow up with their mother relying on them to be, effectively, 'little men'. This has always happened sporadically in history, when men went away to wars, but such responsibility can be a whole lifetime's experience for an increasing number of boys. As single-parent families increase in number, more boys will effectively win the Oedipal battle. This can lead to inappropriate bonding between the mother and the boy, with, perhaps, one or both finding solace in fantasy for what they cannot have in real life.

There are few fantasies that cause my patients more distress than those involving their parents, brothers or sisters, and they take very careful handling. After a great deal of hard work all round, I find that the resolution of the Oedipal material brings harmony to the individual's current relationship in a way that seems miraculous to his or her partner.

Sometimes a fantasy starts off by being attractive and exciting, but ends up by killing desire. I often find that incest fantasies are like this. Here's one woman's fantasy, which illustrates the phenomenon rather well:

FORBIDDEN FRUIT

I have no fantasies normally; in fact, I find it terribly hard to get aroused at all, even with my boyfriend, who's very considerate. Anyway, about two or three times a year I do feel randy, and when I do I start to think about my Dad. When I was little he actually did play around with me. He bathed me a lot well into my early teens and while it felt unnatural and somehow wrong I couldn't stop it. I expect I found it a bit exciting, or I wouldn't be using it now as a fantasy.

It starts off with him bathing me and then towelling me down. This feels nice. My Mum was always very hard and angry, and shouted at me a lot. I never felt she loved me unless I

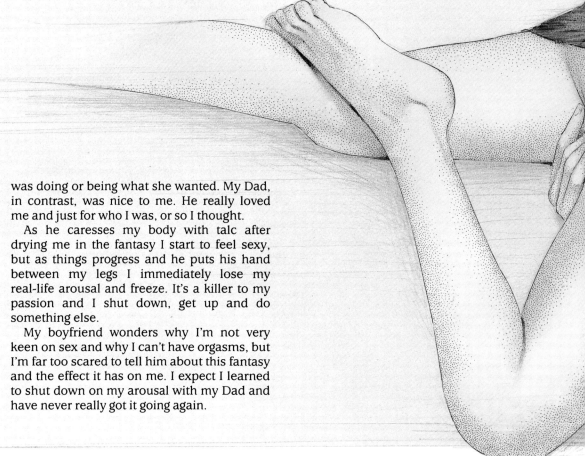

was doing or being what she wanted. My Dad, in contrast, was nice to me. He really loved me and just for who I was, or so I thought.

As he caresses my body with talc after drying me in the fantasy I start to feel sexy, but as things progress and he puts his hand between my legs I immediately lose my real-life arousal and freeze. It's a killer to my passion and I shut down, get up and do something else.

My boyfriend wonders why I'm not very keen on sex and why I can't have orgasms, but I'm far too scared to tell him about this fantasy and the effect it has on me. I expect I learned to shut down on my arousal with my Dad and have never really got it going again.

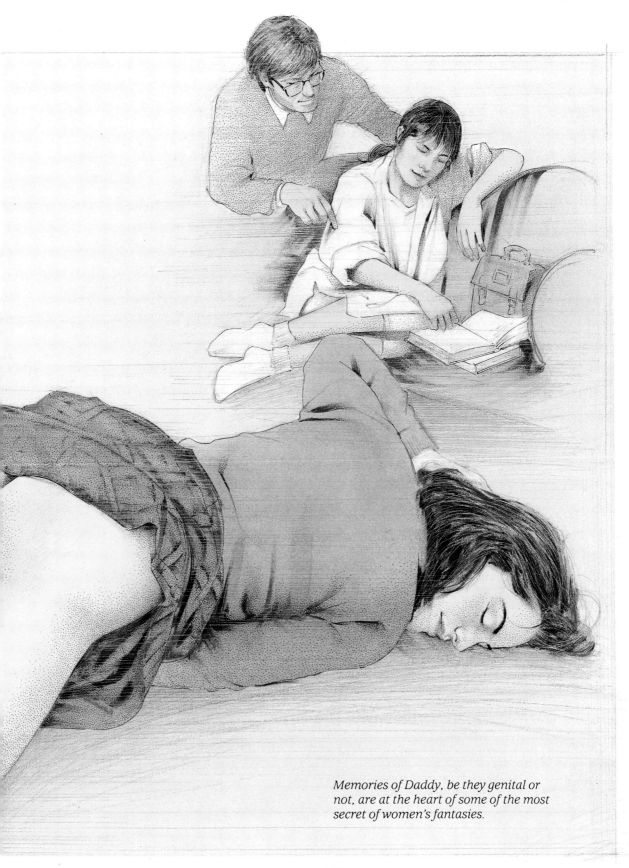

Memories of Daddy, be they genital or not, are at the heart of some of the most secret of women's fantasies.

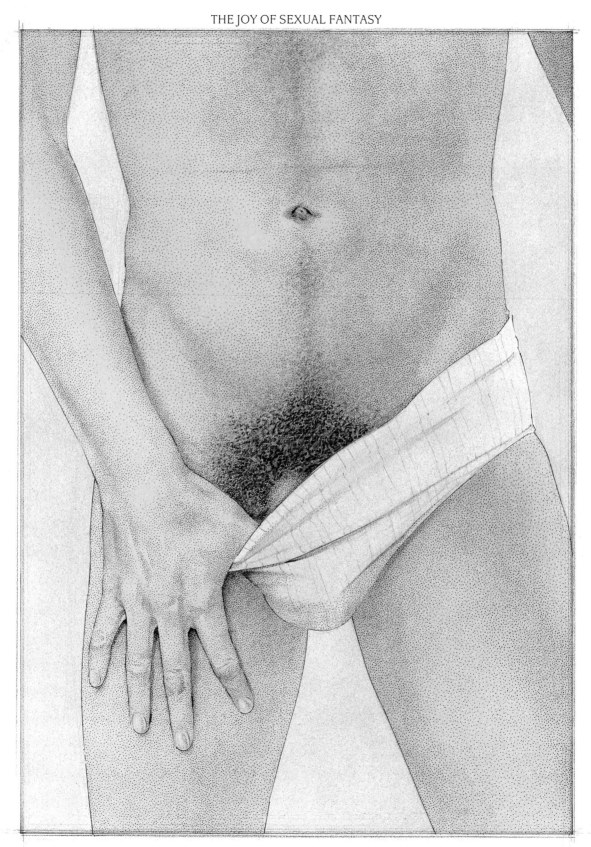

EXPOSING YOURSELF PROVOCATIVELY

Exhibitionism and showing off are discussed on page 103. Exposing oneself provocatively is an extension of this. Teasing the opposite sex is a game that some women play a lot, consciously or unconsciously. There's little doubt that a small number at least are still working through unresolved Oedipal problems. Some of these women learned that being seductive and a tease in childhood brought very tangible rewards in terms of gaining Father's attention and love, perhaps at the expense of Mother. Other women say that they feel unsure of their ability to attract men in real life, but in their fantasies they are very seductive and have no trouble getting the man they want.

The best example of this was told to me by a patient who was just starting to explore her sexuality after many years in an unhappy and unrewarding marriage:

THE TEMPTRESS

I'm out in a lovely red Mercedes sports car. It's open-topped and the day is warm and sunny. I drive along with the wind in my hair, feeling very feminine and sexy, much more than I ever really do.

As I pull up to the traffic lights in this small country town I become aware of a very attractive man in the car next to me.

He turns to me and smiles. I know he's interested in me and means business. The lights change to green and I shoot off, leaving him behind in his less powerful car. However, at the next lights he catches up with me and gives me a meaningful look.

'I'll show him,' I think and, reaching down, undo another couple of buttons on my blouse to expose some cleavage.

As the lights go green I get away quickly and watch him in my mirror following close

He knows that provoking his partner in this way will turn her on. But is his body really as superb as his fantasy tells him?

behind. I thought I'd seen the last of him, but, to my astonishment, just before the edge of the town a pedestrian crossing brings me to a halt and he starts to edge his car right up alongside mine as I wait for a child to cross.

This time I very deliberately part my legs as I wait and then rest my hand on the stubby gear lever and fondle it in a way he can't miss.

I'm away at the lights like lightning and guess he will be far behind me. However, on looking in my rear view mirror I see that he's on my tail. I put my foot down and let the car work for me. Unfortunately, the road is rather winding and I can't go much faster than he. As a result he keeps quite close to my back bumper without much effort.

Starting to panic now, I look for an escape and turn off sharply into what looks like a private driveway. Very soon it becomes clear that it isn't a house, but a small country hotel.

I screech to a halt at the front door and rush in, hoping to find someone who'll help get this man off me. But there's no one there. I run upstairs into a bedroom. Slamming the door behind me, I jump on to a giant four-poster bed and try to hide under the bedclothes.

Within seconds he's in the room, pulling off my blouse and tearing my skirt from me, exposing my bare breasts and tiny bikini briefs. He then makes passionate love to me for ages until I'm so sore we have to stop.

SEX WITH A FAMOUS PERSON

Why are fan clubs so popular? Why is it that so many people, women especially, throng to stage doors to mob their heartthrobs? Is it that so many women have drab, unrewarding lives they have to escape? I doubt it.

Famous people, especially those whose looks and talents single them out from the rest of the population, are seen as sexually exciting and interesting. They are seen in public, on stage or screen, in situations that are larger than life, often with sexual or romantic overtones. No wonder, then, that they become the dream subjects of so many.

Fantasies of having sex with a famous person are simply an extension of this process. In such fantasies the dreamer identifies with them and their lifestyle and, for a while, becomes the sort of person the star might fancy enough to have sex with, given the chance.

Of course, few people know what sort of lover Tom Cruise or Madonna might be in real life. Yet for fantasists it hardly matters. Fans are influenced by what the publicity machine sells, and accept unquestioningly that the object of their adulation would make a wonderful lover. And in a world full of harsh realities and unfulfilled dreams, who can blame them?

Sometimes the objects of such fantasies are not the famous people themselves, so much as what they symbolize. In this way a very ordinary-looking person with an exceptional gift becomes sexually attractive as a result of possessing the gift. It is, for example, the star's piano-playing, the association with his or her subject of specialization, or the racing car, that is the stuff of dreams and fantasies. The person who's famous for the gift may, in a fantasy, be just an appendage, needed for human interest in the context of the music, the expertise, the motor-racing, or the wealth.

As with so many other fantasies, the key issue here is safety. There is no chance of being rejected by a famous pop star, if only because you wouldn't have the opportunity to get into his or her bed anyway. How much more satisfying, then, to have an affair in the mind with the star so that you can make everything go just how you want?

Famous people will always tend to be role models for all kinds of behaviour, not just sexual. This makes them fair game for fantasies, although I must say that most of the public figures I've had as patients are amazed that they are seen as fantasy objects.

PRINCE OF PASSION

My fantasy is quite simple, really. I just love Prince. When I put on his CDs I'm in another world. As I listen I imagine I'm having sex with him while he's singing on stage. I change the scene from time to time, but it's always much the same: he wants me and I have the hots for him. Sometimes I can get really aroused just looking at his poster on my wall and listening to his songs, even without touching myself.

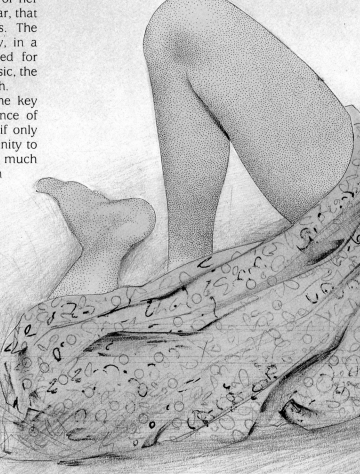

Perhaps it is their very unavailability that makes public figures such a turn-on in many people's day-dreams.

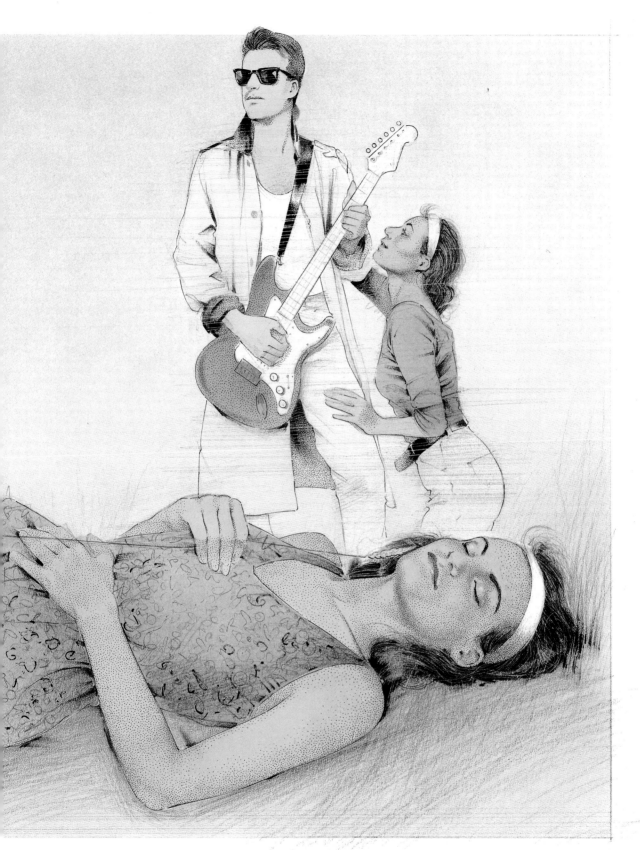

URINATION GAMES

To many people, the notion that urination could have connections with eroticism seems unlikely. Yet there's a large degree of overlap in many people, especially women.

On page 39 I discuss how excretory functions become eroticized in babyhood. This association between the two functions never really dies, but continues to exert itself in many people of both sexes. Because of the close anatomical connection between urination and the vagina, the cross-over remains more powerful in females than in males. Most males understand and accept from an early age that their penis is an organ that carries urine to the outside world. At first this is its only function. But most females have never seen their urinary outlet, so a mystery surrounds the vulva and some women confuse sensations in the urinary system with those in the genitals.

Many perfectly normal women say they get turned on by holding on to their urine. This occurs because the urethra (urinary tube) in a woman is both an erotic organ and a conduit for urine, exactly as in a man. Most people, including a surprisingly large number of doctors, do not realize that the urethra runs in the front vaginal wall and is highly erotic when stimulated. This is probably what the G-spot enthusiasts are talking about. The sensitive G-spot is found along the front vaginal wall. When women are stimulated in this area they experience, at first, a sensation of wanting to pass water. This disappears quite quickly if the woman knows that her bladder is empty. She can now concentrate on the intense pleasure the caress produces and can become highly aroused. The whole urethral area swells during arousal and at orgasm, just as it does in a man. Women tell me that an orgasm induced by stimulating the G-spot feels very different from a clitorally-induced one. They may also leak fluid from the urethra during the orgasm. This ejaculation is not urine, as several carefully conducted laboratory experiments have proved. It is much closer to the fluid produced by a man's prostate gland.

Fantasies involving urinary games – 'water sports' or 'golden showers' – usually originate early in babyhood, when a child's mother showed a considerable interest in bladder function and control. As a little girl grows up, she often finds she can't quite make out which part of her 'down there' feels nice and she may giggle with pleasure as she pees. There's a certain forbidden pleasure about it all which, at this age, she confuses with genital pleasure.

Boys in their early teens who are passing through their 'homosexual' phase of development often play games involving urination contests. It's not uncommon for boys to see how far each can pee in an effort to compete with other males at yet one more level. Given that bigger or further is always better to such thinkers, it's not hard to see how urinary games become yet another way in which a young male can prove his prowess in the sexual arena.

Of course, passing water is a blissful sensation when you're bursting to do so. The sense of relief is not quite parallel to that of an orgasm, but some people, women particularly, claim that it can be close, if only on occasions.

But if all this is healthy and normal, there are other less positive sides to the story. Battles concerning the potty and the dry bed take place in many families and there are few babies and young children who feel totally unemotional about the subject of urinary control. Depending on the home environment and, particularly, on the personality of the mother, a child grows up with varying degrees of negative feelings about, views on, and attitudes toward, urination. A child who is dry can, when the going gets tough at home or at school, regress to bed-wetting as a form of unconscious attention-seeking. This brings the focus of parental concerns and interest back to the child, who has become accustomed to the attention, because after all, Mother was so involved with the subject in the first place. This ploy works. Whatever the child does in the urinary arena creates at least some tension in the mother, who herself has conscious and unconscious views of her own urinary system and its erotic significance.

In adulthood, water sports can serve several purposes. First, they can be a way for a man – and the fantasies of urination games are much more common in men than women – to get back at an over-controlling mother, who forced him to be dry, and put her love on the line to ensure that he was. He might also have a urinating fantasy because it enables him to gain control over his own body. In this sense, the fantasy is less vengeful than assertive.

Last, it might enable him to focus his attention, however unconsciously, on a centre of pleasure that was somehow – although he's not quite sure why – forbidden.

But there is a paradox here, because such an individual is using baby-like regression to assert control or to exact revenge in adult life. What appears to be a sign of power is, in fact, quite the reverse. I like to think of water sports as a way in which an adult can try to get back to the blissful state of babyhood before his mother started to control him and threaten him with a loss of love if he didn't obey her.

Men who fantasize about urinary games often think of passing water over a woman, or even of her drinking it. Urine is sterile and can do no harm if swallowed. Ancient Tibetan and Chinese medicine has always used urine as a curative, but to Western society the notion of swallowing urine is abhorrent. Consequently, most urinary fantasies in which this occurs are, in my view, a manifestation of the individual's anger and rage at his mother and her control. More passive urinary fantasies are probably less driven by anger, as is evident in Jim's story. His is a baby-like fascination for urine and, I believe, a desire to have the woman he loves accept him for his perfectly healthy interest in it. Many women's urinary fantasies are more directly concerned with the naughty links they feel exist between urinary function and genital pleasure. In this sense, I think they're often more straightforward than similar fantasies in men.

Jim is a normal enough man in his fifties. His divorce came through last year and he took up with a woman about ten years younger than himself. After a stormy marriage it was like a haven of peace. When they'd been going out for a few weeks and having normal, pleasurable sex, he started to have this fantasy:

THE SWEETEST SHOWER

I get Jane really aroused and ask her to caress me so that I'm nearly ready to come. I then take her, partly undressed, to the loo and ask her to sit down. I kiss her deeply and caress her tits and as I do so I tell her to pee. She obliges, and as she does I reach down between her legs and bring her to orgasm and feel the lovely warm liquid running over my hands. She comes as she pees and this makes me ejaculate all over her tits. It feels like heaven. I'm totally accepted and loved.

WEARING CLOTHES OF THE OPPOSITE SEX

This is an almost exclusively male fantasy and is not a very common one. In Western culture women are allowed to dress in male-style clothes. In Western societies it was the norm for many hundreds of years for men to wear trousers and women to wear skirts. Now, however, trousers are so commonly worn by women as to be considered a unisex garment. Nevertheless, the association of men with trousers is strong in the West, so they still by and large mark out male from female dress. Women can wear shirts, ties, shoes designed for men, anything they wish. Given that in real life any type of dress is acceptable for women, it's hardly surprising that few women have fantasies to do with dressing in men's clothes.

On the other hand, men aren't permitted to wear dresses, silky underwear or other female apparel, yet such things can be attractive in themselves, and practical in ways that much men's clothing isn't. The taboo on men dressing themselves as women is strong. Priests wear 'dresses' deliberately to make themselves appear sexless – a rare example of men being allowed openly to sport such garments. It's therefore hardly surprising that some men at least have fantasies of dressing in clothes they find sensually or sexually arousing.

The subject of cross-dressing is complicated and the scope of the subject too great for its detailed inclusion in this book. There's little doubt, however, that a few men who indulge in cross-dressing have experiences from early childhood that gave them mixed messages about their gender assignment, but the vast majority have no such conscious memories and simply enjoy the clothes for what they are. The majority do not want to be women, even in the deepest recesses of their unconscious. There is, as would be expected, all kinds of unconscious material that comes to light in therapy with such men. Some don't much want to be men in the classic, cultural, stereotypical sense. Others feel that the feminine side of their personality cannot be adequately expressed in modern society. Very few such men are homosexual; the issue doesn't

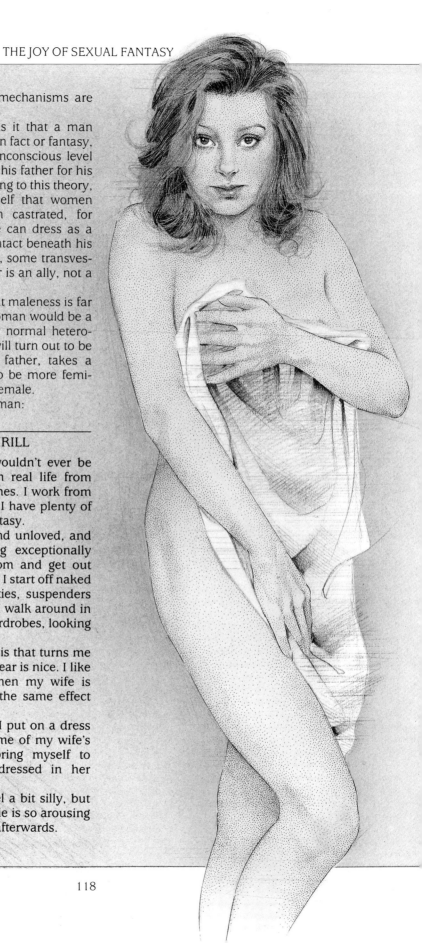

arise and the psychological mechanisms are rather different.

Psychoanalytical theory has it that a man who dresses up as a woman, in fact or fantasy, is deeply concerned at the unconscious level by fears of being castrated by his father for his interest in his mother. According to this theory, the man can reassure himself that women aren't men who have been castrated, for whatever reason, because he can dress as a woman but his penis is still intact beneath his skirt. To complete the picture, some transvestites fantasize that their father is an ally, not a castrating enemy.

Other men have learned that maleness is far too harsh and that being a woman would be a lot nicer. Perhaps a perfectly normal heterosexual male, fearing that he will turn out to be like his tough, unemotional father, takes a more gentle view and tries to be more feminine, while not wanting to be female.

Perhaps Arthur is one such man:

Dressed to Thrill

I'm not a transvestite and wouldn't ever be one, but I do get a thrill in real life from dressing up in my wife's clothes. I work from home and she's out a lot, so I have plenty of opportunity to indulge my fantasy.

When I'm feeling lonely and unloved, and sometimes when I'm feeling exceptionally happy, I go into our bedroom and get out some of my wife's underwear. I start off naked and then put on a bra, panties, suspenders and high-heeled shoes, then I walk around in front of our long-mirrored wardrobes, looking at myself.

I honestly can't say what it is that turns me on, but the feel of the underwear is nice. I like to run my hands over it when my wife is wearing it and it has much the same effect when I feel myself in it.

Sometimes, but not often, I put on a dress and pad out the bra with some of my wife's tights, but usually I just bring myself to orgasm lying on the bed dressed in her underwear.

Afterwards I sometimes feel a bit silly, but at the time wearing the lingerie is so arousing it feeds my fantasies for days afterwards.

SEX WITH AN INNOCENT

For people who are unsure of their sexual personalities, who are socially immature or insecure, or who have little experience with a sexual partner, seducing an innocent holds great thrills. After all, in the presence of a complete beginner the seducer stands to look good. And individuals who fancy themselves as experts in bed can adopt a teaching role and make things happen for the innocent. This can, paradoxically, be mixed in with the insecure type. Men in particular rather like the idea of taking a clean sexual slate and writing their own story upon it. This is why sex with virgins is so popular as a fantasy theme. The inhibited man who cannot face sex with an experienced woman for fear of failure or ridicule will always like the notion of a virgin, but far more often elements of ownership, appropriation and servitude are involved. Some people like to buy a new, rather than a second-hand, house. They say there's something special about being the first to live there. Some men and women feel the same about lovers.

There is, however, also a sadistic element to certain men's virgin-deflowering fantasies. The woman is vaginally small, and immature sexually, and has to be 'made' to take their large organ. Undoubtedly some men with small penises or who fear, however unconsciously, that they aren't well endowed, have such fantasies because the woman's vagina is so small the first time that she will think his organ more than adequate; and anyway, she has no experience from which to judge that it isn't.

Being seduced by an innocent has its own very particular pleasures in fantasy. It is, according to some men, all the more delightful if, on experiencing the fantasy woman in bed, she turns out not to be nearly as innocent as she appears. This has much to do with our

She may look innocent, but once this male fantasy figure is aroused, she becomes a tigress as his sexual prowess transforms her.

cultural prohibitions on female sexual expression. There's still, even in an age of supposed freedom for women to express their sexuality, a considerable brake on women seeming to be too sexually available. Girls are brought up from the cradle to hide their sexual charms, rather than exhibit them openly.

Women have often told me that they consider their best ploy when attracting men is to play down their obvious sexual allure and to appear innocent. That such a kitten then turns out to be a tiger in the bedroom comes as a real joy to the man involved, who kids himself that only in his expert hands could such a transformation possibly have occurred. Such flattery is at the very heart of many male-female dealings, in and out of the bedroom. Consequently, sex with an innocent is and always will be a popular male fantasy theme, as long as the penis and its ability to perform are under question.

SWEET SIXTEEN

In real life I'm a double-glazing salesman. It's a damned good job if you're young and single like me. My fantasy is based on a real event that happened to me one day when I went to this woman's house. I was measuring up for replacement windows when she came in to tell me she was going out for a few moments.

There I am going about my business as usual when I'm disturbed by a young girl, who must be about 16, coming into the room. She introduces herself as the daughter and sits down to chat. I know I'm only 29, but I feel like her dad, she looks so young and innocent.

She starts to talk to me about the job and the people I must meet going around homes. She's seen some video about the steamy life of a door-to-door salesman and asks me if this is the sort of thing I have to contend with.

I tell her that such things do happen, but find myself wanting to play it all down because she's so young I hardly think I should be leading her astray with my raunchy stories of lust behind the double-glazing. I do, in fact, meet a lot of bored, lonely women who are only too ready for a bit of fun.

Anyway, she seems to find my rather throw-away explanation acceptable. She gets up and leaves.

I carry on with the room-measuring and go off down the corridor to the next set of windows. Imagine my surprise when I open the door, to see the girl lying on her bed with just a bra and panties on. I make to leave.

'Don't go,' she begs. 'You can measure anything you like in here,' she says, stroking her firm young breasts.

'You hardly look old enough to know what you're getting into,' I say, trying to back out.

'I'd be a change from the dried-up old women you usually get offered,' she teases.

With that, she crosses from the bed and, coming up close to me, plants a big wet kiss on my lips. I half-heartedly push her away.

'I may look innocent but you can bet your sweet life I'm not,' she taunts. 'Afraid you won't be able to make it with someone young and beautiful like me? Only works with older women, does it?' she teases, grabbing my half-erect cock through my trousers.

This is more than I can take. I push her down on to the bed.

'Get your knickers off,' I order, annoyed at finding myself the mouse instead of the cat for a change. What the hell is this little whore doing? Is she even old enough for sex?

But my concerns are short-lived as she pulls me towards her and undoes my trousers. Pulling out my prick, which is by now gigantic, she admires it like an expert.

'Mmm, nearly as good as those I see in my mate's hard-core vids,' she muses, as she eyes it with glee. 'Get your trousers off and let me feel it inside me before my mum gets back.'

The next part varies according to the mood I'm in. Sometimes I ejaculate before I have sex with her, because it's all so exciting. In another version her mum comes back, finds us at it and joins in. This one gives me my best erection and orgasm as mother and daughter fight over who will have my prick where.

Charles's fantasy of sex with a virgin combines the thrills of seducing an innocent and initiating her vagina, and has sadistic overtones:

VIRGIN PASSION

I've always had a thing about virgins and my favourite fantasy is about this girl I went out with once a long time ago. She was very sexy but I knew at the time she was a virgin. One day we were alone at her parents' house.

My fantasy begins as we get aroused, kissing and cuddling in the den. I get an erection and she's obviously very excited. I say I want to have sex with her, but she says she's afraid because she's a virgin and wouldn't be able to take anything the size of my prick, judging by what she's holding in her hand. I tell her not to worry, but just to lie back and let me look after her.

I slip her panties off and kiss her stomach and thighs for some time. I gently put a finger inside her vagina. She's very small, her opening grips my finger so tightly that the sharp edge nearly cuts my finger off. I keep it in her, and she begins to feel safe and relaxes.

She gets her breasts out of her dress and starts to play with her nipples. I realize this is a good sign that she's excited, so I slowly try to insert another finger into her to stretch her a bit. She obviously finds it painful.

Guessing that I'll need to get things over with quickly, I kiss her very deeply and, while she's totally absorbed, her tongue darting in and out of my mouth with ecstasy, I put two fingers into her as far as they'll go. She cries a little as they open her up, but her body soon settles down and becomes floppy as she realizes that it's going to be OK.

'Are you ready for my cock now?' I ask her.

'No, not yet, stretch me some more with your fingers. It's a monster, you'll hurt me.'

I now put three fingers into her, one above the other. She draws a sharp breath as this forces her cunt walls open even more.

I take a breast into my mouth and start sucking it furiously. She arches her back as she becomes even more aroused. While she's in another world, I sharply turn my whole hand so that my three fingers come to lie across her vagina.

This opens her up so much that she screams out loud and clamps her legs together to prevent me going any deeper into her. I'm afraid someone will hear and I calm her down with gentle talk and kisses, and reassure her.

She soon relaxes enough to open her legs again and, looking down, I notice that my fingers are blood-stained. Without a word I get between her legs and put my cock in her.

She sighs with pleasure as it sinks into her open cunt. 'Deeper,' she begs, opening her legs wider.

And as she takes me right into the heart of her wet, warm body, I ejaculate.

SEX WITH SOMEONE MUCH OLDER OR YOUNGER

Dear old Oedipus is never far away from an explanation of this type of fantasy. Certainly, someone who is older has more experience and more *savoir faire*, but whatever the conscious explanations, most people who have such fantasies are dealing, usually unconsciously, with unresolved Oedipal material regarding the parent of the opposite sex.

Given that incest fantasies are so rarely acknowledged, it should come as no surprise that thinly disguised versions of the same fantasies are found in this category. In Western youth-oriented cultures many people in middle age have thoughts of sex with a younger partner. Males going through the mid-life crisis usually choose much younger females as their playthings, even if only to convince themselves that the young bucks who have bettered them in so many other spheres of life can't have it all their own way.

Today's mid-life woman is also turning to younger men, perhaps on the perfectly rational basis that if she is to choose a new partner after a divorce, she might as well take advantage of the fact that a man of her own age will almost certainly leave her a widow younger than she would wish. A much younger man can reasonably be expected to remain sexually active and available well into her old age.

But this reasoning pales into insignificance compared with the unconscious unresolved Oedipal problems that sometimes colour an individual's past. A father or mother who was over-involved sensually or sexually with a child; a teacher or other important adult figure of the opposite sex; and even *fantasy* adults from childhood or adolescence, all now reappear under the guise of an older or a younger sex partner.

Sex with someone much younger has much the same sort of appeal as seducing an innocent (*see* page 119), but it can also have more sinister overtones, depending on how much younger the sexual object of the fantasy is. Sex with children and really young people is not a common fantasy, except among those who are 'into paedophilia', perhaps in reality. I feel uneasy about encouraging such fantasies in anyone, because turning them into reality is so abhorrent. In my view, those who have such fantasies regularly, or who feel they need to act them out, should seek professional help.

Angie's fantasy gave the final clue that was needed to sort out why it was that she couldn't have sex with her husband, whom she loved very much. In therapy, working through her previously unconscious desires for her father enabled her to function sexually with a man her own age:

THE KNOWLEDGE

Things start in a London taxi. I'm in my early twenties and I'm going off for quite a long ride somewhere on business. It's a very rainy day: the cab's windows are steamed up and I feel very safe, as if I'm in a tiny room. The cabbie is about 60 and is warm and friendly. We talk and he pays me a few compliments.

The motion of the cab and the memories of a really nice session with a previous lover make me feel a bit aroused. I'm often rather like this just after a period – sometimes I feel I can hardly get through the day without sex.

As I slowly get wetter and wetter, this old guy witters on the way cabbies do, but quite pleasantly and in an interesting way.

Then, out of the blue, he says, without turning round, 'There's something in that little cabinet there you might like.'

I glance down to the space between the two flip-up seats to see a small veneered cabinet I've never seen in any other taxi. I open it cautiously to find a vibrator inside. Shocked, I go to close it, but I'm somehow attracted.

'You found it?' he enquires. 'Yes,' I stammer, not knowing quite what to say.

I now start to become more adventurous in my fantasy. 'Hang it,' I think, 'I'll use it. The driver can't see anything and no one else can.'

I slip off my panties and unexpectedly thrill to the shocking coolness of the plastic seat on my behind. I pull up my skirt a little, push my fanny towards the edge of the seat and start to play the buzzing toy on my clitoris. It's not long before I'm ready to climax.

When I'm nearly there I'm aware of the cab stopping. One look out of the steamed-up windows shows that we're in the middle of a park. Before I know it the driver has opened the door and is in the back with me. 'Like me to finish you off?' he asks, kindly.

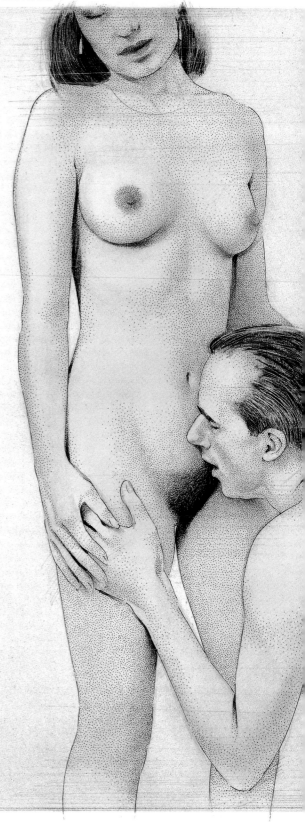

Without another word he takes the vibrator from me and starts to play it expertly over my vulva. Before I can stop myself I'm kissing him as he plunges the plastic monster into me, buzzing parts I never knew I had. I climax time after time as he stifles my noises with his large, sensual mouth.

When he's exhausted me with orgasms using the vibrator, he tells me to get down on my hands and knees on the floor. What follows is the most amazing experience as he pleasures me from behind like I've never felt before. Finally he kisses me tenderly and helps me dress before getting back into the cab and driving me to my appointment.

Hilary's story is of sex with a male much younger than herself:

TOY BOY

Down my road there's a young guy whose name is Tom. I expect he's only about 15 or 16, but he's a real sweetie. He's got this cute little baby face but, at about six foot three, the body of a man.

One day I'm in my backyard, sunbathing, when he comes around to give me a message from his mother, who's a friend of mine. He's embarrassed at seeing me in a bikini and blushes like mad. I try to put him at his ease by asking him to sit down and have a glass of lemonade with me, but he says he has to go.

I know his mom is out, so I tell him that the sun is so good in my private suntrap he should sunbathe for a while with me.

With a lot of encouragement from me, he undresses, leaving only his jeans on.

'You won't get your legs brown like that,' I say, reaching over to undo his belt. This throws him, but I know he really likes the attention, so I go ahead and take his jeans off. The bulge of his penis is now very plain to see. He tries to hide it, without success.

I turn on to my stomach and, undoing the strap of my bikini, ask him to massage my back with suntan oil. I can feel his hands shaking with a combination of excitement and fear as he does as he's told, but it feels good nonetheless and, when I turn over he's look-

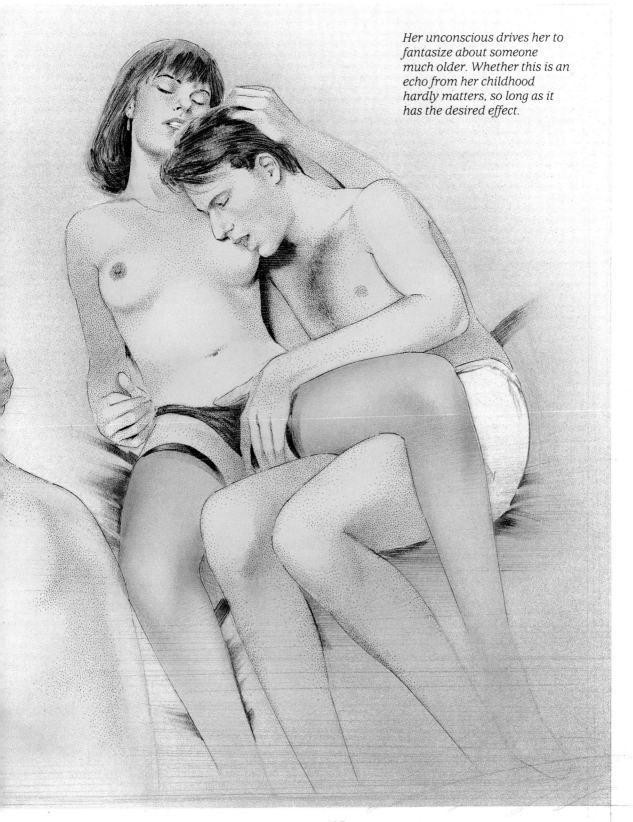

Her unconscious drives her to fantasize about someone much older. Whether this is an echo from her childhood hardly matters, so long as it has the desired effect.

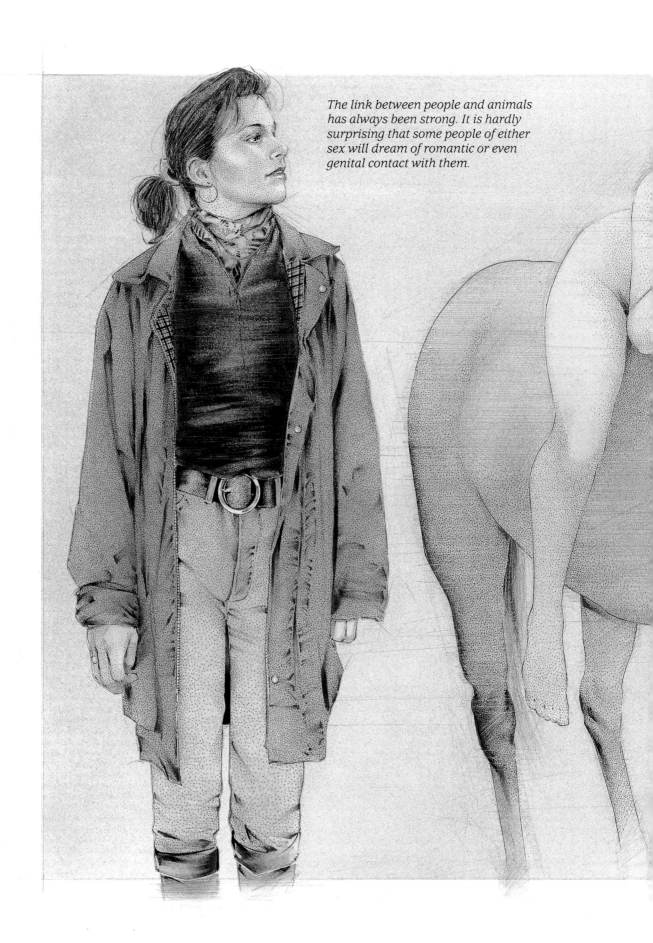

The link between people and animals has always been strong. It is hardly surprising that some people of either sex will dream of romantic or even genital contact with them.

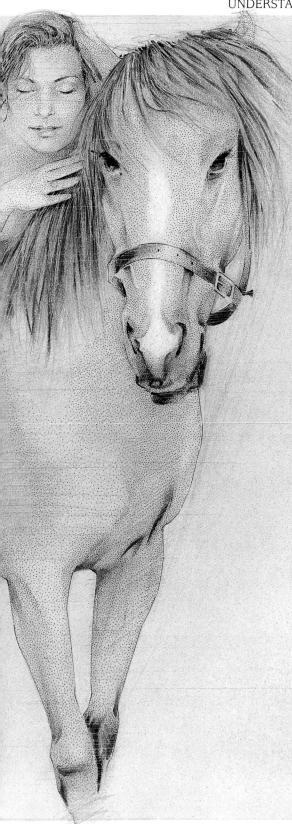

ing like the cat who stole the cream.

Reaching down to take hold of his bulging cock, I ask him if he'd like anything massaged. He says he would, but he shouldn't because his mom would kill him if she ever found out.

'Don't you worry about her,' I reassure him. 'This will just be between the two of us, O.K?'

This seems to calm his fears and he eases off his underpants and lies down on the lounger beside mine.

Slowly, I manipulate his tool to an enormous size. I'd forgotten what a giant it can be in a horny young man. It's clear that he won't last long, so I bring him off quickly while popping his balls between finger and thumb of my other hand.

He's delighted by it and hurriedly makes his excuses and leaves. Once I'm alone again I bring myself to several delicious orgasms just thinking of his young, throbbing prick.

SEX WITH AN ANIMAL

When I talk through women's fantasies with them, there are few topics that arouse more distress than their fantasies of sex with animals. Yet in some surveys this kind of sex comes high on the list of female fantasies.

Sex with animals has ancient mythological origins. The significance of such stories seems to be either impregnation and the creation of an offspring with particular virtues, or the heightening of sexual pleasure. Either way such notions are deeply embedded in the collective unconscious all over the world.

Every permutation of sex with animals is depicted in detail on Egyptian tomb paintings, but with the coming of the Talmudic code and the Old Testament, sexual intercourse with animals was prohibited. Since then zoophilia, as the practice is technically known, has been taboo in almost every Western culture.

Nevertheless, all kinds of bodily and sexual contact between humans and animals takes place, much of it between males and animals kept as pets or on farms. Kinsey, in his study, found that about half of all males brought up in rural areas had had some genital contact with animals. Female activities with animals have always been less common in real life.

In fantasy life, however, it is my experience that sexual contact with animals is more common among females than males – but I don't practise in a rural area. Such fantasies, as described by their originators, usually involve a domestic animal, often a pet which has almost as much emotional significance to them as have their human acquaintances. For some women, the fact that the animal takes them over in their fantasy and makes them climax absolves them from the guilt of making things happen. One of my patients had repeated fantasies of her German shepherd dog licking her to orgasm after real-life experiments in which she encouraged him to do so.

Some people resort to such fantasies after disappointing real-life experiences with humans. They retreat from the trials and tribulations of sex with humans and dehumanize the process. Individuals who have other kinds of fantasies involving non-human objects or participants also dehumanize their sexual arousal. Males who have such fantasies say they can get an animal to perform many more exciting sexual games with them than their partner would or than their experience of human partners tells them any other person would. Some people claim they fantasize in this way only when depressed or going through a period of sexual deprivation. They say that this sort of powerful, yet non-human fantasy protects them from affairs and extra-marital dalliances when they feel tempted to indulge in them.

Power and control are central to human sexual interactions. Some people who use animal fantasies say they completely do away with both of these issues in their sex-with-animals fantasies. There's no ongoing commitment; and no bargain to be struck, as in real-life sex, or even fantasy sex, with a human. Fantasy sex with animals is pure sensation, with no fear of having to pay an emotional price. For some women, who have a poor view of men and do not wish to play the cultural role required of them, fantasy sex with an animal has considerable attractions.

For women there is possibly also another factor. Those women with whom I have discussed this say they love their pet, and that it loves them. This caring and loving relationship can, they argue, develop into a sexual one, and then perhaps even a genital one. Women of all ages complain that they obtain too little unconditional love, yet, they say, their domestic pet seems to love them just for who they are. This, they argue, is the basis for real love. And real love can easily justify real sex.

People leave their money to their animals, bury them in cemeteries and reorganize their lives to feed, mate and exercise them. There seems little reason to believe that their emotions are any less involved – and they are not. Some women say they would be more upset by the death of their pet than their husband.

As with the majority of such unusual fantasies, the owner would not want to act them out. From the points of view of hygiene, personal safety and cruelty to animals it would probably be unwise to.

STANDING TO STUD

My fantasy came directly from a book by Nancy Friday. Of course, I've changed it to be just right for me, but it's a bit like her story about the woman being fucked by a donkey.

I love riding in real life. In fact I like almost everything about horses. I've seen a stallion in a field weeing, and watched in fascination the gigantic penis elongate and then go back to its former size. I've seen mares being mated, too, and the sheer size of the horse's prick arouses me.

My fantasy is about being captured by a band of gypsies in the heart of the countryside. They take me to their camp and parade me half naked in front of all the young men. One of them has a birthday and I'm to be his present, to do what he likes with. He decides I will have sex with his favourite stallion.

I'm terrified of what will happen, but have no choice as the young men grab me by force and take me to a sort of large table. I'm then blindfolded and become aware of a crowd gathering. There's music and rowdy noise.

Next thing I'm aware of is that someone is smearing slimey stuff all over my cunt and bottom. I struggle to get free from the bindings they've used to secure me to the table, but can't budge an inch. Within seconds I'm aware of a huge, hot body behind me. It arches over me, me putting its front legs on the table over my shoulders.

The young man whose birthday it is now reaches down to the horse's prick and, whispering tauntingly in my ear that it will be the biggest thing I've ever felt in my life, helps the animal's throbbing penis into my vagina.

As it enters even the tiniest bit it hurts fit to kill me. As the gypsies see me writhing in agony and terror, they start to sing and chant.

The young man now encourages the horse with coaxing words and, as he does so, its vast penis rips into me, making me scream uncontrollably. I'm sure it will tear my insides to pieces as it starts to thrust in and out and as I climax, I faint with the agony of it.

SEX WITH SOMEONE OF A DIFFERENT RACE

Although early observers of sexual fantasies reported this theme to be fairly common, it is not my experience today. I believe that the unconscious drives to have sex with a black man, for example, are much less in evidence today, when coloured people are no longer a novelty in Western countries.

Only 20 or 30 years ago I think quite a few white women felt a conscious and unconscious attraction to black men in particular. They were said to have enormous penises and to be able to satisfy a woman like no white man could. This in itself was enough to make them attractive subjects for female fantasies, given that many women have reveries involving very large organs or sex toys that stretch them and give them exquisite pelvic sensations of being filled up.

Not only did the fantasy black man have a prize penis in the unconscious of many women, he was also a prohibited character in many conservative white societies, bearing all the ancient and taboo associations with all things black. Given that the unconscious of many women is littered with dark notions of sexuality, including its sinfulness, it is hardly surprising that at least some women will use a black man to symbolize this forbidden material. If a white woman has problems with her parents' views of sex being forbidden, how much better to give them one in the eye, even if only in fantasy, with a man they would find more unacceptable than a white man?

For white people today, much of this notion of the mysterious and exotic black has lost its fantasy power, as millions of whites and blacks all over the world meet and marry. However, there's still a fascination for the foreign. I see this most in women – although it's also sometimes found in men – who want to take a rebellious stance against parents, society or whomever. In therapy, such matters provide useful insights along the tortuous road that leads to fantasies about sex with someone of another race or culture. To some individuals, sex is permissible only in the context of such foreignness. In a sense, it is a little like sex with an animal or a sex toy, in that to some extent it removes the sex object from reality and somehow dehumanizes it.

Some fans of this type of fantasy say they wouldn't indulge in such activities in real life. In this sense they are laying old and probably unconscious ghosts by dealing with 'strange', 'foreign' people in their sexual fantasy. Many people use dreams and fantasies to cope with the anxieties that such material raises and with which they can deal in no other way.

Liz's fantasy is a good example of many of the points raised here:

THE THRILL OF THE UNKNOWN

I'm white and I live in an area populated largely by blacks. I meet lots of black guys at work and some of them are quite attractive. But I've never been turned on by any of them enough to do anything about it.

But my fantasy involves two black men. One night I'm on my way home from work quite late when these two guys come out of a soul music store and start to flirt with me as I walk. I try to brush them off, but they're insistent. They suggest going to a club just around the corner and I find myself interested because I like the music played there.

In a few minutes we're there and the place is throbbing with the beat. I love that deep rhythm, it does something inside my cunt.

The two guys now suggest that we dance and they take turns to dance with me – ordinary dancing, not smoochy or close.

'Want to come backstage and meet the band?' one of them asks.

'Yes,' I reply, eagerly.

'Come on then,' he shouts above the din.

We go backstage and stand right next to the performers in the wings. I'm starting to get a real buzz from the smells, the excitement, the sheer pleasure of it all. 'These guys really know how to enjoy themselves,' I think, as they start another number. 'Can I meet them afterwards?' I ask.

'Sure,' he says, 'Come with me.'

I follow him hesitantly because we start going into the dark bowels of the building.

'In here, Whitey,' one says, pushing me into a tiny dressing-room. The other one slams the door shut behind me.

'Take your jeans off,' the first one orders.

I'm dumbstruck. 'No way,' I splutter defiantly. Now the whole adventure suddenly turns nasty on me.

Not used to being crossed, the first guy comes straight over to me and, taking me firmly by the waist, rips open my jeans and yanks them and my panties down my legs.

'Kneel down,' says the second one, taking out his prick, which is starting to get bigger. 'Suck on this, white girl. Like a bit of black sausage, do you?' And so saying he thrusts his prick at my mouth.

While all this is going on, the other guy goes behind me and holds my hips. He brusquely forces my legs open, pushing my feet apart with his foot. Suddenly he's in me with a cock the length and thickness everyone expects of a black guy.

But his friend in front of me isn't getting what he wants. This is all about to change. He reaches down and takes hold of my nose, gripping it firmly. Unable to breathe, I gasp for air, only to find my wide-open mouth suddenly filled with the biggest cock I've ever dreamed of. It thrusts right to the back of my throat, choking me. He lets go of my nose and starts to thrust in and out.

I think I'll die as these two enormous black cocks poke me from both ends. It feels for all the world that they'll meet in the middle around my belly button. The one behind me now reaches round to grab my tits and as he holds my nipples tightly I come and come as each man shoots his semen into me.

MASTURBATION

Masturbation, alone or with a partner, can be used in fantasy by those who are too inhibited to take sexual activity through to its conclusion as sexual intercourse, or as a part of a more complex fantasy.

Mutual genital pleasuring is popular and there's nothing intrinsically inhibited about it. Most such activity, however, culminates in some sort of sexual intercourse or copulation, so it's not an end in itself. In masturbatory fantasies the owner usually finds that masturbation (either way round) is all that can be managed. There's nothing wrong with this, of course, but it can sometimes mean that other areas of sexual life are, for the fantasist, less interesting, free and fulfilling than they might otherwise be. There are those who tell me that such fantasies – tame though they may be – are infinitely preferable to any other.

Fantasies of mutual masturbation are common, as an end in themselves or as a passing delight on the way to more arousing events.

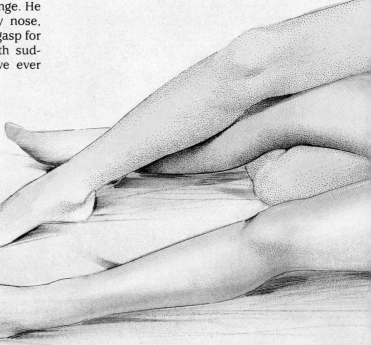

DOUBLE BILL

This fantasy of mine is simple, not like those I've seen in books or sexy magazines. It consists of me and my girlfriend going to see a raunchy film. Some way through I realize she's breathing rather heavily. I put my arm round her and she moves towards me in a way that means she feels sexy. I let my hand go to her lap and to my delight she opens her legs a little. This gives me the signal I need to feel her thighs under her skirt, and very soon she's wide open for me to stimulate her clitoris. I can easily get my fingers around the edge of her panties.

As I hold her she watches the film and I bring her to orgasm. It just ripples through her in a quiet sort of way but I know she loves it.

I take my fingers out of her panties and she brings her knees together, turns to me and gives me a little peck on the cheek. 'Thank you,' she says. Then in real life I ejaculate.

SEX TOYS

These objects have been around for thousands of years. The orientals used carved dildoes and similar things, and every culture throughout history has found ways of enhancing sexual pleasure by using gadgets and potions of various kinds.

Today, with life-long marriages, lasting an average of 52 years, many couples seek to enhance their bedroom games, if only from time to time. The growth of the sex toy industry is legendary: if sales figures are to be believed, there's hardly a household anywhere without some sort of sexy toy, even if it amounts simply to some lingerie a couple uses on special occasions.

Sex toys can be used by an individual for

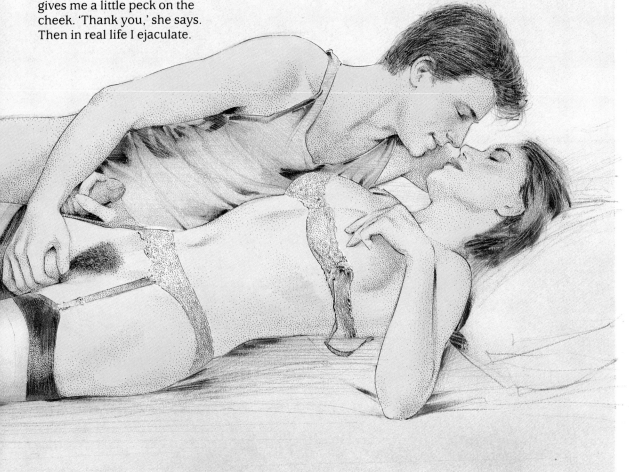

personal pleasure in the absence of a partner; instead of a partner when emotional and other troubles in the relationship make love-making difficult or impossible; or by two partners together. Many women day-dream about their vibrators or dildoes, or use them during masturbation, and for a few women, sex toys form an integral part of their love life.

It's said that men are keener on such toys than women, but this is not my experience. Women may take a little persuading at first, on the grounds that women in Western culture are not supposed to bring about their own seduction, but once this initial barrier is down, things usually go very well. Indeed, given that many women are not sufficiently satisfied by their men, it is hardly surprising that some at least seek pleasure during masturbation by using some sort of aid. The majority of women do not use commercial sex aids, but rather improvise with domestic objects, such as fruits and vegetables, candles, hairbrush handles, shower heads and other objects. There can be few women who have never experimented with such a toy, even if only from time to time and in a fairly low-key way. Obviously it makes sense to be very cautious about what is inserted into the vagina or the rectum. By and large it's best to stick to commercially-produced aids that are made for the purpose.

At the other end of the scale are women such as Anna, whose best fantasy revolves around a present her perceptive husband gave her for her birthday. Her fantasy is based on an event that once took place and it is this event she recalls every time she uses it during a day-dream, or when masturbating:

DIRTY DANCING

Chris and I are going out to a formal dinner-dance at his firm. It's a really big day for him and I'm nervous. He's keen for me to look nice for it, so I buy a flattering new dress. The skirt is very full and when I twirl round on the dance floor I show a lot of leg. I'm a bit of a show-off in real life and like to tease, so in my fantasy I just take this a bit further.

People tell me I've got a good figure. My bust is big and the dress shows off my boobs to their best. I know this turns Chris on, especially when he sees his bosses eyeing me and wishing they could screw me.

It's the evening of the dance and I'm feeling great. It's just before my period and I'm always hot then. We're about to leave the house when Chris comes back into our bedroom with a small, gift-wrapped box. He leans over and pecks me on the cheek and hands it to me. I'm a bit flabbergasted because he often gives me things, but never just before we go out.

With some excitement I open the box to discover a soft rubber thing, which I gingerly unwrap. It turns out to be a pair of rubber panties. But that's not all. As I unfold them I discover that inside there's a dildo the size of a man's erect penis fixed on to the front part.

'Stand up,' Chris whispers in my ear, 'and lift up your skirt.'

I do so, becoming pretty aroused at the thought of what he's going to do. He then slips my knickers off, leaving me standing there naked from the waist down, apart from my black stockings and suspenders.

'Open your legs,' he commands, as he spreads my thighs a little. My feet part easily, even though I'm wearing very high heels. He then reaches for the latex panties and, getting down on to his knees, slips my feet one at a time through the legholes. Quickly and deftly, he pulls them up my legs and when he gets to my crotch tells me to open my legs more. He slips a couple of fingers into me and feels that I'm soaking wet.

Before I know where I am, he has slid the dildo into me and pulled the panties up firmly around my waist. I give out an involuntary cry and catch my breath as the firm latex forces the dildo inside me.

'There,' he says, 'that should improve your dancing. Now let's get going.' With that I let my skirt fall and we're on our way.

When I sit in the car the feelings are quite amazing. I can feel the movement and vibration of the car deep in my vagina, in a way I've never experienced before. When this all first happened I nearly had an orgasm before we even got to the dance.

As soon as we get out of the car, we're caught up in a mass of people going into the dance.

As Chris warned, dancing with a new toy is quite something else. The sensations are out of this world. Doing the twist is best, as I swing my knees from side to side and crouch down. The best part of all is when I'm dancing with Chris's boss, who has always wanted to get me into bed. 'If only he knew,' I think.

When Chris and I dance together he asks

me how the dildo feels inside me and we give each other knowing looks as I cautiously sit down for the first time, taking most of the weight on my feet.

As the evening wears on I'm starting to get so aroused that I have to have an orgasm and I tell Chris so. He knows I must be almost out of control by now and takes me off to another part of the hotel where there's a bar that is completely empty and in darkness.

We kiss passionately and deeply and he runs his hands all over me, caressing my breasts in the way he knows I like. Slowly and very tenderly, he lifts me on to a bar stool. As he lets me down, the dildo goes deeper into me, because, with my feet off the ground I'm unable to take some of the pressure off it by bracing my feet.

Chris leans forward over me, kisses me deeply again and, while his mouth is on mine, he reaches down and caresses my magic button till I come and come for what seems like ages.

I can never think of this occasion without having an orgasm almost on the spot. It's my favourite fantasy when I wear the latex panties on my own sometimes to bring myself off.

OBSCENE PICTURES AND VIDEOS

This is a complicated category because it contains all kinds of mixed fantasies from many other groups which have been put in the context of porn in one way or another. I find that individuals – male or female – who have such fantasies usually consume large quantities of porn, albeit of a very soft variety. They then put themselves in the picture, so to speak, as if they were creating the porn, or were an actor in it. Clearly this is a way of allowing oneself to engage in sexual activities that would otherwise be unlikely, impossible or even undesirable in everyday life.

STAR OF THE SHOW

In this particular fantasy I'm an actress in a porn video. It's all rather surreal. I'm taken into a studio where there's a large couch, like a gynaecologist's couch, with stirrups for my legs to go up in. A faceless man leads me to it

and secures me on top of it by my legs and arms. A stout leather strap is then passed over my belly and pulled very tightly around the back of the couch so my stomach and pelvis are completely immobilized.

Now all the lights go down and several men come in. They take seats around the edge of the studio and spotlights are shone on to my body. I feel so terribly exposed – they can see everything. My breasts are open to their gaze and my crotch is on display. I feel so utterly open, I can hardly bear it.

The next thing that happens is that a gorgeous guy enters the room, totally naked. He comes over to me and starts to play with my nipples. He sucks them till they ache, handling my breasts gently but firmly.

As he goes down on me I'm aware that the whole couch starts to rotate. We're obviously on some sort of platform. As soon as this happens, several enormous video screens light up all around the studio. Each shows a different view of my body. There must be a dozen close-ups of my breasts, my mouth and lips, my legs in their stirrups, and two or three different angles of my cunt and behind.

The man now starts to tongue my clitoris, which makes me want to come in seconds. I'm aware that the watching men are also taking part in their own way. I can just catch a glimpse of some of them jerking off as I go around, and I hear a good deal of heavy breathing going on not far from me.

The effect of the guy tonguing me, and seeing every part of my body in such detail on the screens is unreal. Now he puts his prick inside me and starts to pump in and out.

As I'm about to climax again he senses it and takes it out to tease me. When I've cooled off a bit, he plays with my tits some more and then puts his prick back in me. I can no longer bear the excitement.

I open my eyes briefly to see my body in giant close-up, being ravaged by the prick on three large screens. I've never seen my cunt being stretched by a cock before. I've never seen the length of a man's prick disappear into the depths of me and like magic re-appear, only to thrust itself straight back in, right up to the balls.

Orgasm follows orgasm as I alternately close my eyes in ecstasy and open them to see what it all looks like on the surrounding screens. In the background, 12 penises are spilling their seed.

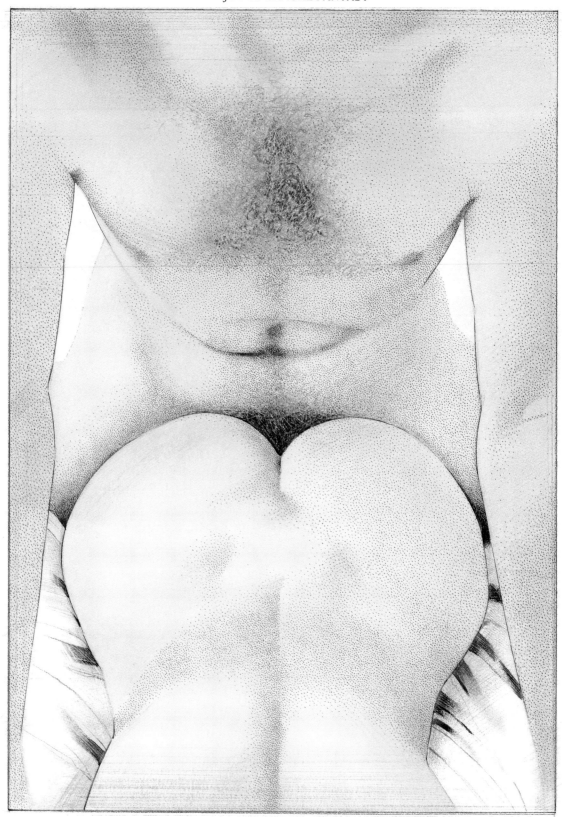

No word passes between anyone during the whole procedure, so it's with some shock that I hear the man who has just fucked me say, 'OK, who's next?'

ANAL SEX

This is a subject that raises all kinds of strong emotions, whether it's dealt with in fact or fantasy. There are millions who, influenced by Judaeo-Christian taboos, reject anal sex out of hand. However, for very many more, anal eroticism has a part to play, both in real life and in the imagination.

That the anus is an erotic zone cannot be denied. Although many people of both sexes don't find it so, my clinical experience is that people who most vociferously deny their anal eroticism are the ones who eventually come to value it most highly. The power of the unconscious over anality is great.

The subjects of toilet-training and early infantile models of anal concern among mothers are too complex for detailed discussion here. Suffice it to say that most people have at least some notion, however unconscious, of their anal eroticism – even if it is only that there is something vaguely bad about it.

Most people, while having some notion of anal eroticism, associate anal play with dirt and forbidden practices. Women seem to have more of a problem with this because they're taught from an early age that nice girls are clean. This is certainly not true for boys, who are allowed to be dirty in every sense of the word, literal and metaphorical. Consequently, males generally have much less trouble with dirty eroticism, compared with females.

Anality is greatly suppressed in Western woman, but men seem to be more at ease with this area of their anatomy. Many women grow up to think of their vagina as a smelly drain. Yet men love it, want to put their fingers and other things into it and even want to kiss it. This creates severe confusion in many women of all ages, who find that what they most fear – smelly holes – men most like.

Anal sex has always been, and always will be, a favourite for a substantial minority of real-life lovers. For them, and for some others who do not actualize their anal desires, anal fantasy is highly arousing.

A lot of men want more anal play than they get. Many a man, given permission, will say that he wants his partner to caress his anal area or even to penetrate him. For the man who sees penetration as a sign of homosexuality, this can be distressing, but millions do not make such an association, they simply enjoy anal sex for what it is.

Women's aversion to anal matters is a bone of contention in many otherwise successful partnerships. When a man loves every bit of a woman's body, he can't for the world imagine why it is that she doesn't return the compliment. Such a man is ripe for anal fantasies.

For some men, whether in real life or fantasy, the demand that their woman participate actively in anal sex with them has far wider implications. Given that it is seen as the most dirty of all sexual activities, it can be used as a test of the relationship. 'If she really loved me she'd want anal sex, or to stimulate me anally,' is how the argument goes. Such a man then makes an issue of this to test how much his partner really loves him.

Some such men even push it to the point of no return and make it a make-or-break issue in the relationship. The latter occurs especially when a man, however unconsciously, wants to break up his partnership on other grounds.

For many men, the ultimate sign of female sexual abandonment is the woman who says, in effect, 'Take me any way you want. All my orifices are yours to use as you will. My body is hungry for your penis.' This is the stuff dreams are made of. And this is why anal sex is such a powerful tool in men's fantasies.

Similar considerations lie behind many women's use of such fantasy material. I find that a women who starts to use anal fantasy is not far off incorporating anal play or even anal sex into her real sex life. Anality is often the last barrier to fall as she lays siege to her sexual inhibitions over the years.

Many women have told me that throwing off anal inhibition is one of the best things they ever did. They look back and see how 'tight-assed' they were and tell of how opening themselves up to their anality revealed more free sexual expression than they had ever thought possible. This may not mean that they ever experience anal penetration. Rather, they come to accept the anus as a highly erotic area. This acceptance helps them put aside childish prohibitions that were having deleterious effects on their sexuality.

Arthur's fantasy illustrates the common male plea: 'Love me, love my anus':

THE DEEPEST LOVE

I'm sure I'm not a homosexual, but I do like my anus stimulated during love-making, and I enjoy my wife putting a finger inside me as I come off. But my fantasy is much more exciting than this and makes up for the fact that my wife doesn't play with my anus in a way I'd really like. She usually makes a scene about doing it at all. Obviously in my fantasy I make it all just how I want it.

There's a woman I work with, who I find terribly sexy. Her name is Sue and she isn't at all available because she's happily married. In fact I know her husband. But this doesn't stop me thinking how great it would be to have her in bed. I don't just go for normal sex with her, though. My fantasy involves her making love to me while I'm almost totally passive. I could never do this with my wife because she needs me to make things happen all the time.

So I'm in bed with Sue and she's coming on strong, running her naked body all over mine as I lie on my back. She reaches down between my legs and caresses my balls. Before I know it she's between my legs, firmly stroking the thick root of my prick. This gives me a deep and wonderful sensation inside, like I've never had before. 'You seem to like that a lot,' she observes. 'Perhaps we should see why it feels so good.'

She takes a small tube of lubricant from the bedside and covers her fingers with it. 'Open your legs wider,' she bids me.

I do so. I'm aware of her finger teasing around the rim of my anus. It's pure heaven. I feel totally open, so relaxed yet deliciously tense, wondering what she'll do next.

Slowly and gently, she inserts first one finger and then two. I feel myself stretching to take her fingers and soon she's seeking out my prostate gland and massaging it. This produces sensations quite unlike anything I've ever experienced, yet strangely, it gives me only a small erection.

'I'm sure we can do better than this,' she says, grasping hold of my awakening prick. Taking it into her mouth, she starts to flick the top slowly with her tongue. Next she runs her tongue around the tip, as if it were an ice cream. 'This is very yummy,' she says, as she takes it out of her mouth.

I almost scream with pleasure as she replaces it and sucks me at the same time as caressing my G-spot deep inside.

As I approach orgasm all my pelvic muscles tense up to become almost painful, so full do I feel inside, but the penis sensations and the prostate caresses send me sky high and I ejaculate just as she pulls her mouth off me and allows my spunk to splurt all over her face. I buck and arch like a wild horse. Sue's hand inside me is unbearably stimulating and my innermost magic spot is tender from her stroking.

She takes her hand out and cuddles up next to me holding me tenderly. 'I love you,' she whispers. And I fall asleep in a state of bliss.

BISEXUAL ACTIVITIES

I explain on page 101 how it is that most people experience at least a tinge of same-sex attraction, if only from time to time and perhaps only deeply in the unconscious. It is but a short step from this to bisexual activities: sex with people of both genders, perhaps even at the same time.

Every personality combines both masculine and feminine character traits. Society expects an individual to express largely one or the other. This means males have to exhibit largely masculine characteristics and females largely feminine ones. However, in the human psyche matters aren't this simple. As a result of childhood experiences, people grow up to own and display various combinations of characteristics along this masculine/feminine continuum. And they may show up in different ways and situations at different times. So a male social worker might, as a caring professional, display his feminine side by being caring, nurturing, loving, compassionate and selfless at work; and then show highly masculine personality traits in bed with his partner. The same goes, in reverse, of course, for a woman.

In bisexual fantasies, I believe people make love to the various parts of their own personality, coming to terms with their need to give and receive, to penetrate and be penetrated and to be active or passive, regardless of gender or usual sexual orientation. To be a receptive male is not necessarily to be homosexual, just as to be a penetrative female is not to be a lesbian.

There are signs that people are becoming more accepting of this blurring of the old cultural stereotypes in which men had to be men and women, women. As these boundaries become less defined out of the bedroom, people are allowing themselves to enjoy the fruits of both sides of their personality in bed, too. Many men today talk to me of their tenderness, their caring, their desire to nurture, their non-competitiveness in bed, their wish to enjoy a pleasurable sexual process rather than a fraught journey toward a sexual end. Ten years ago few men admitted to such feelings. They would have been thought of as latent homosexuals, which they feared more than anything.

For the individual, particularly a man, who has bisexual fantasies, real-life experiences of bisexuality will probably be out of the question, given current fears about AIDS. Bisexuality in the real world was, until recently, growing in popularity, especially in Australia and in the USA. The AIDS epidemic in these and other countries has made many men think twice before making their fantasy a fact. In this sense, fantasy has come to their rescue, as it often does in other areas.

Linda's fantasy is an example of bisexuality in a woman. She feels safe with it because it involves two people she loves and can trust; her husband and her best friend:

THREE-WAY-LOVE

My husband and I have been together for 20 years and I love him a lot. We have a smashing sex life and I've never been tempted to stray. My fantasy is about a particularly sexy girlfriend of ours, Sandra, who we've both known for many years. She has just started to get a divorce.

One day she comes round to our place pretty drunk. Her husband has been giving her a rough time and she has walked out on him in desperation. My husband is kind to her, puts his arm around her and comforts her. We all have a cup of coffee and talk about her problems. She asks if she can stay the night with us and, of course, we agree.

After some time talking we go to bed. I see her into our spare room and settle her down. I give her a peck on the cheek to soothe her and put out the light.

Imagine my surprise when, in the middle of the night, I sense that a third person is in bed with my husband and me. It's Sandra.

'I was so lonely and miserable I couldn't sleep,' she cries, and she snuggles up to me.

'That's OK,' I say, rather taken aback. I put my arms around her and cuddle her like a baby.

'Mmm,' she purrs, 'that's nice. I can't remember when anybody last cuddled me like this.'

I start to rub her shoulders and before we know where we are she's kissing me and stroking me all over. I never wear anything in bed, so this makes things easier. It isn't long before we're both naked, enjoying one another's bodies.

This is all new to me because I'd never had the slightest idea that I'd like to have sex with a woman. Still, I reason with myself that this is hardly real sex – more a sort of cuddling.

In the middle of all this, my husband wakes up. 'What's going on?' he asks.

'Sandra's terribly upset,' I answer.

'We can't have that,' he replies. 'Let her come in the middle.'

I pull Sandra over my body to lie between us.

Jim now starts to caress her, too, but much more sexually than I had done. She melts in his arms. It must have been years since she had sex, poor cow.

I suddenly realize how turned on I'm getting. As Jim caresses her breasts and kisses her firmly and confidently on her lips, I begin to touch her cunt. It's warm and wet and obviously near to an orgasm.

I throw back the bedclothes, get over Sandra's open legs and start to tongue her hard, waiting clitoris.

Jim stops what he's doing and leaves me to kiss her tits and clitoris in turn. This drives her wild and had much the same effect on me.

'Fuck me now,' I say to Jim, as he watches in disbelief his wife bringing their best friend close to a climax.

He moves behind me and thrusts his prick into me. Even though my mouth is full of Sandra's labia, I still make an audible noise. I reach out for her tits to hold. I pull on her nipples and keep working on her with my mouth. She's about to come and so am I.

'Faster!' I cry out to Jim and as he rams it deeper still inside me, I start to climax.

Sandra, feeling this, lets herself go too, and with a throaty sort of scream begins her own orgasm.

We girls have several orgasms before I feel Jim push deeply into me in a way I know means he too has come.

We all fall into a heap, cuddling one another, content and sexually relieved.

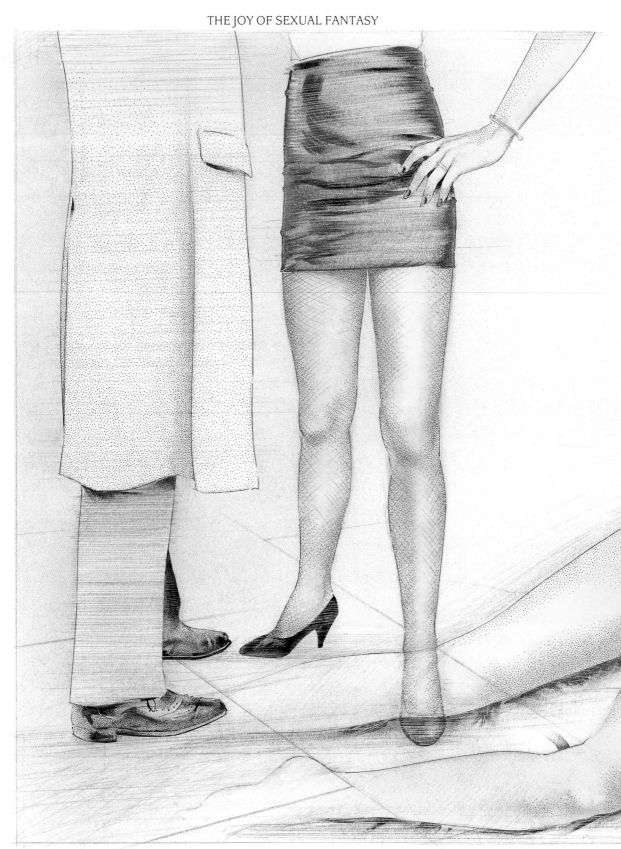

BEING A PROSTITUTE

In my clinical experiences this mainly female fantasy is usually enjoyed by women who are rather inhibited sexually in their everyday lives. In this type of fantasy they indulge their true sexual selves under the guise of being paid for a service. I sometimes find that women start to have this sort of fantasy as they become more aware of their sexuality. They experiment in fantasy with their new sexual discoveries as if they were a child let loose in a toy shop.

Although this woman would never want to be a real prostitute, it helps her arousal to imagine she's so sexy that men will pay for her favours.

Prostitute fantasies not only allow a woman to engage in all kinds of activities she wouldn't otherwise enjoy but they also enable her to have sex free from the commitment to a partner. It's sex for sale; sex at the impersonal level; sex for its own sake without cost or entrapment; sex as a commercial commodity. And, some women say, it's a chance to show off.

For those women who have had poor experiences with men in real life prostitution can be a very attractive fantasy. It can also be very flattering, as one of my patients told me. Unlike her partner, who was rather unadventurous and boring, the men in her fantasy wanted her to do all kinds of exciting things. Moreover, she got paid for it.

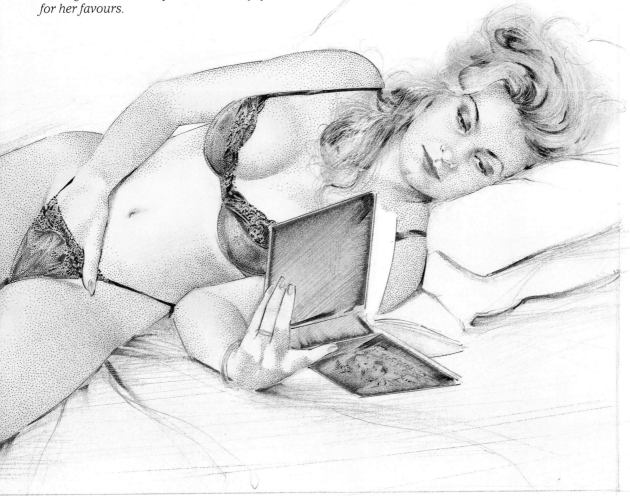

FIVE FINGER EXERCISE

In my fantasy I'm a prostitute in a high-class brothel that costs the earth for men to visit. I do this as a part-time job to make more money for our family. I go there several afternoons a week and I'm the star turn. All the regulars ask for me. I'm known for my expertise and the men pay a lot extra to have sex with me.

On this particular day a very important man comes to the brothel. 'Julie,' says the madam, 'I want you to take especially good care of this gentleman. He's over here from the USA and is missing his wife terribly.'

I take him to my room, where I undress him caressingly. 'Anything special you want?' I ask, cautiously.

'Sure is, honey. I want to watch you come.'

'Is that all?' I ask in disbelief.

'You bet,' he replies.

'OK then,' I say as I stretch out on the bed.

'You come over here and sit by me.' I then lie back on the luxurious silk sheets and start to play with myself.

He's obviously excited because I can hear his breathing quickening as well as mine. He doesn't touch me at all, but just watches as I become more aroused.

I play teasingly with my nipples after taking them out of my bra. I slip my hand down around my cunt and caress myself. I pull my panties to one side and slide a finger or two inside my vagina, in and out, to arouse myself and to turn him on.

'You sure there's nothing else you want to do?' I ask, fearing he might complain if I do everything for my pleasure alone.

'Take your panties off and I'll maybe finger you as you come,' he says, sounding excited.

I expertly remove my black silk panties and throw them across the bed. Lying there with my legs wide open, I feel him open my labia and insert a finger. This feels good, so it isn't long before I restart my self-stimulation and begin to lose contact with what's happening around me.

As I become more aroused I'm aware that he's inserting another and then another finger into me, until I think I'll burst. But the stretching makes me so wet and horny that I know I'll come very quickly.

He sees this and, wanting to prolong his pleasure, removes his fingers. I gasp in frustration.

'Put them back, please,' I beg.

'Sure will, honey,' he purrs and so saying, gently but firmly pushes his whole hand into me. I have never, in all my experience with men, felt anything like it. It's as though my whole pelvis is exploding, but it's totally and mind-blowingly exquisite.

Not content with just having his hand in me, he starts to rotate it back and forth with his fist clenched. This catapults me into excruciating orgasms, the like of which I've never known. As I climax time after time he keeps rotating the hand till I nearly faint from the painful ecstasy of it all.

At this point in the fantasy I always come, but sometimes I carry on and think of him leaving me a really big tip as he leaves. It's funny, but sometimes after masturbating to this fantasy I actually do get a sore cunt.

DOCTOR-NURSE

This fantasy is usually seen in men, who, despite radical changes in the profession over the last two decades, persist in imagining all nurses to be women. However, there's a female variant of the fantasy, which involves caring for a man.

A sexual fascination with female nurses dates from the days of Florence Nightingale and the very start of the profession. These women, it was hinted, would answer more than just the medical needs of their patients. And, ever since the profession was founded, some nurses have sought and given sexual pleasures in the course of their job. In this they are probably a little different from any other group of people dealing with the opposite sex at work.

Nurse fantasies arise from several sources in the conscious and unconscious. First there is the very obvious caring behaviour. When they go into hospital, people regress to childhood in many ways. The surroundings are strange and induce fear; the reason for being there produces yet more unease; and some of the time patients have to undergo painful or difficult procedures that make them feel even more like children. It's a situation of dependence and vulnerability.

It should come as no surprise, then, to find that many people look up to female nurses as a type of mother figure. This is usually fine for most female patients, but for men it can produce emotions that are unconsciously linked to their own mother and her caring behaviour, or lack of it, when they really were children. It can also reactivate old Oedipal cravings.

A combination of vulnerability, feeling like a child and having a woman perform often quite intimate rituals on him can all too easily confuse a man into reading things into the relationship that aren't there. After all, many men are inept at interpreting man-woman relationships. Dealing with personal bodily functions also brings back memories from the unconscious – memories of other significant females doing the same things in the past.

Given that many men have unconscious confusions about such matters, as is evidenced throughout this book, it's hardly surprising that sex and nursing go so frequently together in men's fantasies.

Many men tell me that their current partner doesn't care for them very well or very much. By 'care for' in this context, they mean 'minister to them lovingly'. The contrast in hospital when a female nurse, even though she is paid to do it, looks after their personal needs so effectively, can cause confusion and genuine lust, because it is lacking in their lives.

In certain situations, which will be part of the experience of some of the men who have such fantasies, a man will have spent quite some time with a nurse in a setting which, under other circumstances, would have led to intimacy and even sexual activity. For example, a man who, when ill, is in the company of a nurse for many hours a day, perhaps with her sitting by his bedside at night, when things are quiet, can easily find not only real caring at the professional level, but far more. In fact, a few nurses have told me how close they can become to certain patients (of both sexes) over a short period of intensive time together.

Another point is that when a man is in hospital his normal sexual life comes to an end. If he's well enough he will be able to masturbate, but there are almost always unmet sexual needs in such situations. In fantasy he can have sex with the females who are there, and those he sees most of are the female nursing staff.

Some men's fantasies of nursing situations verge on the passive. The female nurse is in charge, has to do something to him she would otherwise not do socially, and then finds while

she does it that he is sexually exciting and irresistible. The desire many men have for sexual novelty means that nurse fantasies legitimize their raunchy thoughts in a way that isn't usually permitted. After all, there are few other situations in life in which a man might legitimately be undressed or be so personally ministered to by a woman. Nurse fantasies cut straight through all these social barriers.

For the man who likes pain (and perhaps has masochistic fantasies), nursing procedures that create discomfort can provide just the right sort of balance of pain and eroticism. She has to do it because it's her job, yet he can tolerate it because she's so sexually attractive.

Yet for all this a nurse is supposed to be untouchable. She's only doing her job. The man with such a fantasy wouldn't have such overt sexual thoughts about a bus conductress or a woman selling lawn mowers. This very untouchability makes nurses all the more exciting as fantasy material. In the mind of the fantasist, nurses are allowed to do what they want to their male patients in the name of duty, but the man himself isn't allowed to do anything. This is the very meat of good fantasy material, whatever the setting.

Some men tell me that sexy things really have occurred in their hospital experiences. Understandably, such episodes are incorporated, alongside other details from real life, into the fantasy.

Alan's story illustrates very well just how erotic a fantasy about a female nurse can be. It's loosely based on a real experience he had when in hospital for a hernia repair in his teens:

A DOSE OF LOVE

My fantasy starts with my favourite nurse coming in to change my dressing a few days after the operation. She's tall, has the most gorgeous hair and a beautiful figure. I've been eyeing her for some days and get a hard on just thinking about having sex with her.

On this particular day she comes into my private room. After closing the curtains to make the place completely private, she pulls down the bedclothes and says she wants to look at my wound to see if it's healing well.

Slowly she opens my pyjamas and pulls them down to reveal my groin. The smell of her body, the way her hair glistens in the sunlight and the presence of her so close and

*An old favourite with some men. Will it become
a powerful fantasy for women, as male nurses
become more commonplace?*

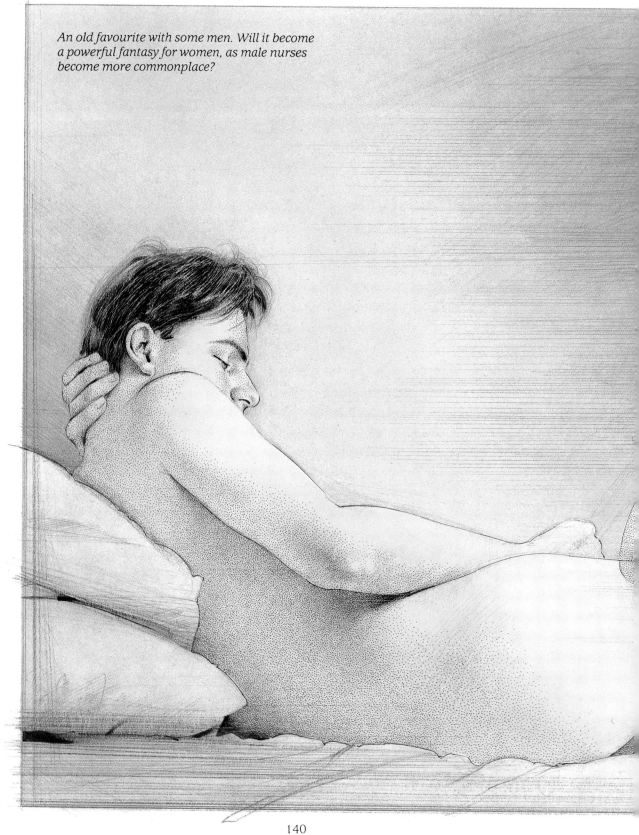

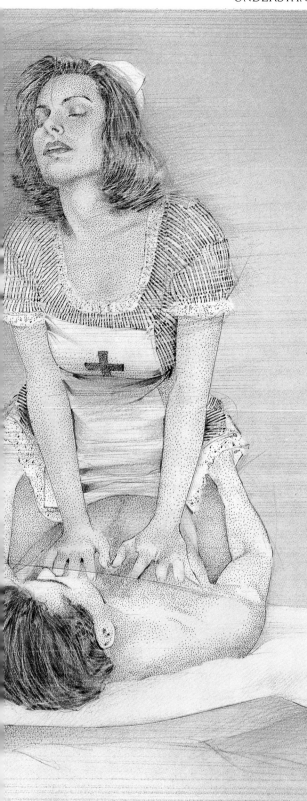

yet so far, make me feel really horny.

She starts to inspect the wound and, as she does so, I begin to stir. I pretend not to notice because I'm so embarrassed, but it's all too obvious what's happening.

As she finishes replacing the dressing, she 'accidently' brushes her hand against my penis, stirring me into action even more.

'I think we'd better check that this still works all right after the operation,' she says, taking my penis into her hand and massaging it to produce an enormous erection.

'Seems perfectly OK to me,' she whispers as she sees the effect she's having.

Then without more ado she bends down and slips it into her mouth. I'm flabbergasted, but delighted. She then fellates me as expertly as I imagine any woman could and within seconds I'm panting and ready to come.

'Hold on,' she murmurs, after taking my red, throbbing prick out of her mouth, and goes over to the door and locks it.

Before I know what's happening, she raises the skirt of her uniform and kneels on the bed astride my penis. I lift up the starched material to see that she's wearing black stockings with lacy tops and nothing else. 'The bitch,' I think, 'she came here ready to fuck me. I'll show her.'

Being careful not to disturb my hernia wound, she lowers herself on to my prick and moans with pleasure as its swollen head stretches her cunt opening. I'm virtually immobile because I'm lying down and because, frankly, I'm scared to death to do too much in case I burst my stitches.

'This should take the pressure off your groin and let the wound heal,' she whispers as she moves rhythmically up and down.

I reach under her starched white apron and fondle her breasts. She caresses herself.

Just at that moment someone knocks on the door. It's the head nurse wanting to come in.

'We won't be a moment,' my nurse calls out in a stifled voice and, within seconds, she shudders with her orgasm and I shoot into her wet pussy.

Without saying a word she gets off me, covers me up, straightens her uniform and leaves the room, pausing only to give me a backward glance and a satisfied smile that I shall remember for the rest of my life.

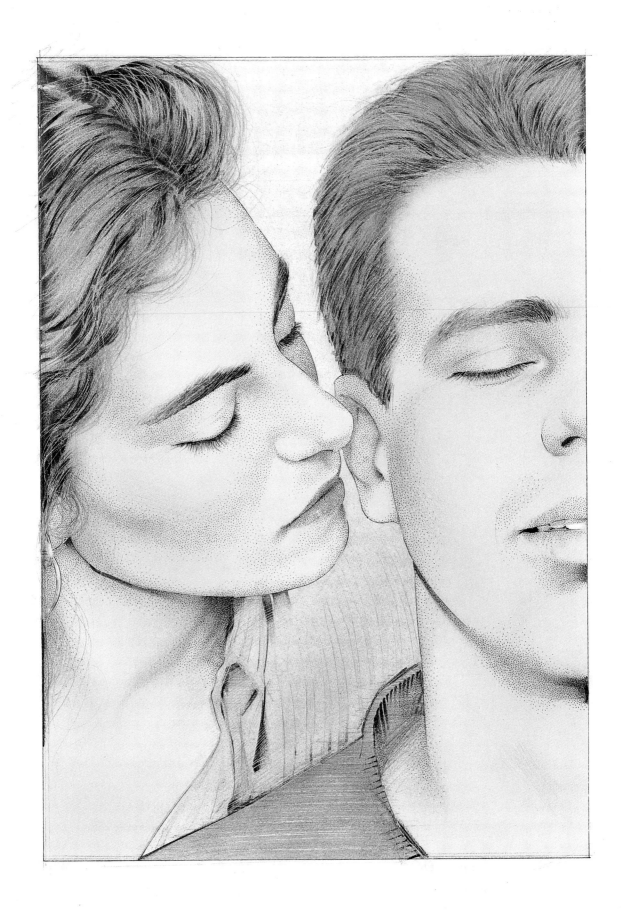

PART THREE

How to Fantasize

Some people claim to be unable to fantasize at all;
others to fantasize only in a very limited way; and
there are yet others who fantasize readily and freely,
but find it hard to know whether or not to share such
fantasies with their partner. These subjects are all
considered in the following pages.

Fantasy is an almost universal experience in humans, as Part One shows. Yet I often come across people who claim they never fantasize. While I believe them when they say this, I don't believe they are incapable of fantasizing, given some help. Indeed, it is my clinical experience that those who say they don't have sexual fantasies often eventually discover that they do, but that the subject matter is so unacceptable to them that even before it reaches consciousness it is censored. In this way they can honestly say that they don't fantasize.

Getting past such a block can call for professional help, but this is often not necessary. It is perfectly possible to learn how to develop your ability to fantasize. I take my patients through a teaching programme and many are amazed at how proficient they become over only a very few weeks. If you want to learn to fantasize, you can teach yourself to do so at home.

At the heart of learning to fantasize is the ability to visualize mental pictures. Some people are more visually orientated than others and find this easy. Others find it very hard because their main sensory way of working is perhaps tactile or verbal. It's always worth starting with visual images, though, because with practice they can produce excellent results that will encourage you to add in other things as you become more skilled.

There are seven steps to learning how to fantasize. How long each step will take depends on how much time you have available to practise; your starting point; your unconscious; your conscious 'brakes'; your will to do it; and much else besides. Work through one step at a time, progressing to the next only when you have mastered the existing one. Take your time.

STEP 1: RELAXED BREATHING

Make a time and space for yourself in a quiet place, where you won't be interrupted. Make sure you're warm. Take the phone off the hook and lie down on the bed, sit comfortably in an easy chair, or lie on the floor – whichever enables you to feel really relaxed.

Close your eyes and take some really deep breaths in and out. Breathing in the following way will be really relaxing: take a deep breath in so as to fill the top of your chest with air. Immediately let it out in a way that makes your whole body go floppy and relaxed. Once the breath has left your body, either through your mouth or nose, immediately breathe in again right up to the top of your chest. Once you have the hang of it, this circuitous breathing without stops produces deep relaxation within only 20 or so breaths.

Don't breathe in this way for more than a few minutes. Once you feel nicely calm and relaxed, you're ready to start on Step 2. With practice you will be able to get to this calm, relaxed state within a few minutes of starting the breathing.

STEP 2: IMAGINING A SCENE

As you lie or sit pleasantly relaxed, try to imagine a scene of some kind in your mind's eye. It is easiest at first to re-create a scene that you have witnessed. Many people like countryside or seaside scenes for this part of the procedure. If you want to be really sure of success, start by visualizing your garden or a favourite room.

New places for sex, especially those with an element of 'danger', are real winners. Making love in a car has particular value in this couple's shared fantasy life as they re-live their courtship days.

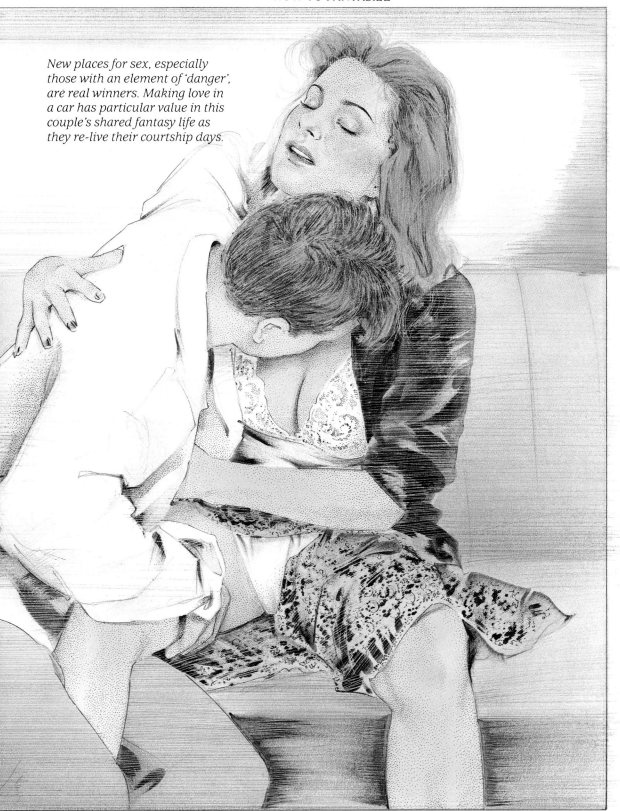

Just quietly picture the scene in your mind's eye and become aware of what's going on. Slowly extend the scene from a static, postcard type of image, by embroidering in some detail. What colour is the sky? Are there birds? Are there other people or are you alone? What colour is the sand? Are there flowers in the field? Ask yourself other questions. After a few minutes of doing this you should be able to 'see' your familiar scene quite clearly. Stop there. Open your eyes, allow yourself a few moments to come to, then go about your daily tasks.

Repeat this process several times over the next week. Each session need only take a few minutes, but as the days go by you will find that you will able to get into your scene quicker and that there will be more and more detail in it.

STEP 3: IMAGINING YOUR BODY

Get yourself nicely relaxed, as in Step 1. When you are ready take yourself through the following exercise. You will need to be lying down for this step.

Imagine that, at your feet, some height off the ground, is a large reservoir of a warm, honey-like fluid. It is going to run via a tube into your body through your feet. Concentrate single-mindedly on your toes. Feel the honey filling them up. It is warm and heavy and makes your toes warm and heavy as it fills them up. Take yourself through each toe in your mind's eye and feel it filling up with the warm honey.

When you feel your toes are warm and throbbing with the honey, allow it to fill your lower legs up to your knees. Just picture it flowing up towards your knees. When it has reached them and your legs feel warm, relaxed and heavy with the honey, continue on to fill your thighs in the same way.

Next, let the honey flow into your pelvis and fill up your stomach to the base of your chest. This is also a large cavity and it takes a long time to fill. Feel the warmth of the honey not only inside your stomach but also in its walls. Now allow the honey to flow into your chest and, if you are female, your breasts. This is also a large volume and takes some time to imagine becoming full.

When your chest is full up and the whole of your body from the neck down feels heavy, relaxed and warm, allow the honey to overflow into your arms, right down to your fingertips. Once this is complete, take the honey up through your head to the very top of your skull.

Your whole body should now be warm, relaxed and heavy with honey. Stay with the feelings and relish them. After a while open your eyes. You will feel deliciously relaxed and calm.

I have made this sound easy and for some people it can be. For others, though, it can take some days of practice before they can easily feel relaxed and full of warm honey. Don't get discouraged if you can't achieve this in the first few sessions. Keep at it. Concentrate deeply on the feelings of warmth and heaviness and you will be surprised how quickly you can drop into this kind of deep relaxation.

STEP 4: COMBINING STEPS 2 AND 3

The next stage in learning how to create erotic fantasies involves combining what you have learned from Steps 2 and 3. In this stage you get relaxed as before, preferably lying down, and then when you are totally full of honey, completely relaxed and warm, create your favourite scene as you did before, with your eyes closed.

The combination of profound relaxation and the pleasant scene should open new possibilities for you. You will probably find that your sensitivity to the scene is far greater than it was and you should, with practice, be able to imagine things that your other senses would pick up if you were really in that scene.

Try to hear the sounds, smell the smells, feel the textures and so on as you work your way around your scene. One woman I did this with recently was able to describe and sense the texture of the leather, the smell of the coffee, the perfume she was wearing and much more besides, in a railway carriage that formed the basis of her scene.

This step takes a lot of practising, but with perseverance you will be able to get good at enriching the scene you started with, so that it really comes alive. Be prepared for this to take several weeks. As you become more adept, you'll find that you'll be able to drop into your favourite scene without the breathing, the honey or even the relaxation. At this stage you'll be able to do it on a train, while waiting for a bus, while doing the gardening, or whenever you choose.

When you are happy that you can not only see things in your mind's eye but can also feel them, you are well on the way to being confident of creating sexual and erotic fantasies.

STEP 5: YOUR FIRST EROTIC FANTASY

Start off by fantasizing about something simple that you know turns you on. Perhaps read a sexy magazine or part of a book, or watch a suitable video. If this is too difficult or intimidating, just imagine a sexual encounter that you have experienced. I find that this exercise is usually best done after a period of relaxation, as described in Step 1 (*see* page 144). For the best results fill yourself with warm honey first as in Step 3 (*see opposite*).

Once you start creating your erotic scene, keep it simple, non-threatening and rewarding. Try just imagining a loving event between you and your partner, if you have one. Keep away from genital activity at first, if you want to. Simply imagine cuddling or being cuddled. As you become more at ease with the process of creating a fantasy you'll be able to extend the sexual activities to become more adventurous and, eventually, genital. If at any stage you feel anxious, stop. Go back to the part of the scene where you felt OK and stay with that. When you have enjoyed the scene for long enough, bring it to an end.

STEP 6: YOUR SEXUAL BODY

This is a really interesting and exciting step. It used to be said that the only way people could become sexually aroused was by experiencing some sort of sexually arousing stimulus in their environment. The sex gurus Masters and Johnson wrote nearly 30 years ago that a man cannot create or will an erection. This is not so. Both sexes can, with practice, create quite high levels of sexual arousal simply by thinking about sex or something specific that arouses them. This is the most difficult stage of fantasy training and will call for all the skills you have learned so far.

Get deeply relaxed; fill yourself up with honey and imagine a sexually interesting or exciting scene. All of this should come quite readily to you by now if you have done your 'homework' regularly. Now imagine a new source of hot, as opposed to warm, honey flowing into your body. I will look at each sex in turn because the details of the visualization differ, according to whether a male or a female is doing this.

If you are a woman, start off by imagining your breasts getting larger, warmer and fuller, to the point at which you can really feel the hot honey filling your breasts and nipples, so that they feel tense and throbbing with hot honey. Take yourself on a guided tour of your breasts, experiencing the feelings of the hot honey expanding them, and your nipples becoming tense and erect. When your breasts are full, throbbing and hot with this honey, imagine it spilling over down your stomach to your genital area. Feel it filling your vagina, your outer and inner lips and, finally, your clitoris. Take your time visualizing this, just as you did with your body filling with warm honey ear-lier on. Get the hot honey to fill up each part of your genitals and feel them swollen and hot. As you get good at this you will find that you start to lubricate and that your clitoris will swell.

Over some sessions of practising this technique you will discover that you can become aroused in fact,

This fantasy is popular with men who want or need to be somewhat passive from time to time. He just lies back and enjoys having things done to him.

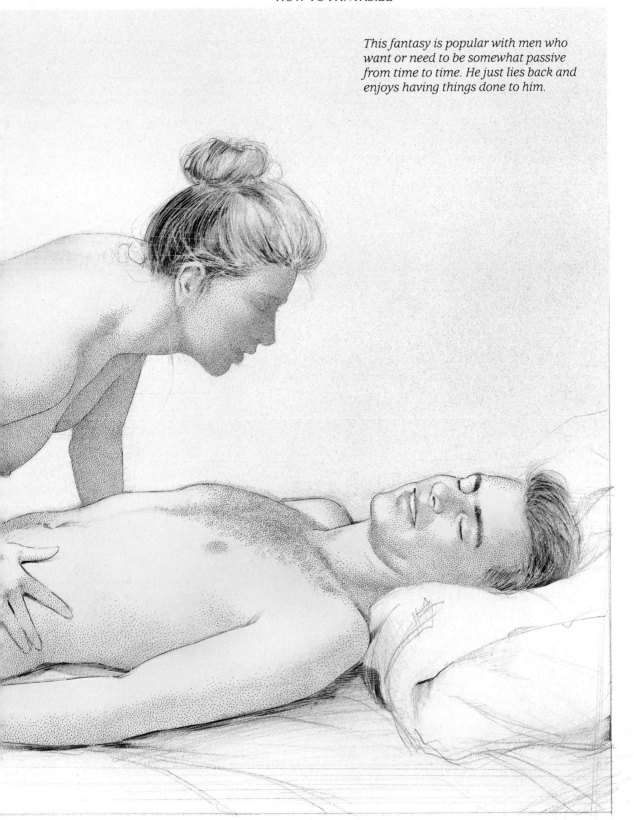

149

not just in your mind. With perseverence and enrichment of the images you should be able to create a pleasant feeling of arousal that might make you want to masturbate.

If you are a man, start off by imagining hot honey filling your scrotum. Feel your testicles enlarging and pulsating with the hot honey. Really concentrate on them filling up and becoming large and heavy. Now imagine your penis filling with hot, enlivening honey. Feel it getting thicker, longer and hotter. As you do this, if you concentrate really effectively, you will find that you can get an erection even if it isn't a full one. Practise until you can will some sort of erection by this visual imagery. The erection you obtain may not be a full one but you will be aroused and could then 'convert' it into a usable one if you want to have sex or masturbate.

STEP 7: COMBINING STEPS 5 AND 6

You are now nearing the end of your fantasy practice. In this final stage, start off by creating sexual arousal using your hot honey technique, and when you are really aroused and feeling deliciously excited, start to add in your favourite sexy scene. The two together should have a highly arousing effect and you will probably want to make love or masturbate, depending on the circumstances you find yourself in at the time.

Lastly, practise this so that after some weeks or months you will be able easily to drop into both the bodily and psychic components of your imaginary scene. This is the heart of erotic fantasy. Gradually, over some weeks, you should be able to do away with more and more of the training props (the breathing, the relaxation, the warm honey and so on) if you want to. The real 'pro' can become sexually aroused simply by using his or her mental picture.

My experience of taking many people through this technique proves to me how effective it is. Repetition is the key to success, though this takes some patience in the early days as new skills are learned. Perhaps the greatest problems come as things progress to the stage where people find that they cannot think what scene to picture. By definition this can be a difficulty for the individual who has never fantasized. I suggest that you look at any source of sexy material you have ever found attractive. Most women find that romantic stories arouse them, but for many, a men's magazine with its erotic stories and pictures is even more effective.

Men by and large find visually explicit material best. This is why most males learn to masturbate to pictures of naked or near-naked women. It used to be said that women weren't as aroused by visual erotica, but as females in our culture become more aware of what they most enjoy, it is clear that this old myth applies to a few women only. Similarly, rather than always having to have everything laid out on a plate for them, some men really do enjoy romantic and other less overtly genital stories, which give scope for their imagination to fill in the missing parts.

Reading a book such as this should give you a feast of ideas for erotic fantasies . . . indeed, over the years I have used Nancy Friday's book, *My Secret Garden* (Quartet 1976), as a way of helping patients obtain new erotic fantasies to add to their existing bank, or to create them if they have none.

As you start to learn how to let your unconscious have its head, you may well be surprised at what comes up. A story that a few months ago might have revolted you could now become highly arousing. A sexual scene previously unthinkable in reality (which was all you had) can now be accommodated with great pleasure in fantasy. You may also find that you start to dream erotically for the first time, as your unconscious takes the brakes off. Trust your dreams and go with them . . . in fantasy at least.

One woman who I took through this process was quite near the end when she had a very exciting, if alarming, dream. She was the main girl in a high-class whorehouse. She was dressed the best of all the girls, taught them what to do to please the customers and was renowned for her sexual expertise. In the dream she loved this adulation and felt sexually very strong and confident.

One day a tall, fair American man came to the establishment and said he wanted her. She offered him all the other girls, but he was adamant. She was flattered because he was such a turn-on.

Just as she was warming to the idea and trying to be suave and highly professional in front of the other girls, he announced that he wanted her to have anal sex with him. She was deeply shocked. She was overcome with confusion, lost her cool and refused to do what he said.

'I'll do anything else you ask,' she told him.

'I know you will,' he replied, 'And that's why I'm going to make you do something you won't do – have anal sex.'

At this she woke up in a blind panic yet highly aroused.

As we worked through this dream, she started to incorporate the idea of anal eroticism into her imagery practice and surprisingly, to her, found that she enjoyed it hugely. It wasn't long before anal pleasures formed a major part of her sexual repertoire, both in fantasy and, later, in fact.

Another way of discovering new topics on which to fantasize is to write the outline for a sexy X-rated video which you are to direct. One day, when you are feeling good, get relaxed, perhaps have a small alcoholic drink, get yourself a little aroused and settle down to write a highly sexy script outline. As it will never be acted out you can be outrageous. Make it as exciting and detailed as you can. You will be surprised how erotically creative you can be.

DEALING WITH GUILT AND ANXIETY

For those who have always fantasized and who find that fantasies flow easily from somewhere they can't pinpoint, guilt and anxiety are usually only a problem when the material that surfaces is hard to accept. I looked at this in more detail on page 32. When you are learning to fantasize from scratch, though, there is a greater likelihood of guilt and anxiety rearing their heads because you are so obviously and consciously trying to create sexy scenes that make you aroused. This, I find clinically, makes more women feel bad than it does men. Older women, especially, still tend to see sex as something they have little control over and for which they are not responsible. Such women tell me that the conscious act of creating erotic scenarios makes them anxious before or guilty afterwards, however pleasurable it is at the time.

There are no simple answers, except perhaps to say that if you find this a problem, try to go gently and to keep within the bounds of what your internal censor can cope with. Some women I have helped find that they are fascinated by some of the more outrageous things they read when exploring the idea of erotic fantasy, but cannot include such topics in their own personal fantasy life, at least not at first. I suggest going slowly with much less threatening subjects, and gradually working up to more complex and difficult topics as time and confidence progress. A partner with whom you can share any of this can help greatly. I look at this in more detail soon.

Just as you can desensitize yourself to anxiety and guilt in real life, so is it possible to do this in your fantasies. Let me take a simple example. Supposing you find you are excited by the thought of taking your man's penis into your mouth and bringing him to orgasm, but that it creates anxiety while you are fantasizing and guilt afterwards. Both get in the way of your pleasure. Here's how you can get over guilt in the fantasy.

Start off in real life by dividing up your problem into ten separate steps. Here are some suggestions:

1 Touching my vagina after my man has made love to me. I feel his semen.
2 Semen leaks out of me on to my thighs as I lie on the bed after sex.
3 He ejaculates on to my tummy.
4 Kissing my man's penis in the dark.
5 Taking the whole head of his penis into my mouth.
6 Doing the previous two in the light.
7 Taking the whole penis in to my mouth and moving it in and out.
8 Kissing his scrotum.
9 Bringing him near orgasm in my mouth, then letting him ejaculate on me.
10 Bringing him to orgasm in my mouth.

When you are somewhat aroused one day, start off by visualizing a scene which involves only your Step 1. Really enjoy it. Revel in it and, if you are totally happy with it, take the story a step further. When you arrive at a step that makes you feel anxious, stop. You'll know that anxiety is creeping up on you because you'll become less excited. Go back to the previous stage and masturbate to orgasm thinking of this. At the last moment, as you come to a climax, you may be able to go one step further up the ladder without loss of excitement or anxiety.

Repeat this process over a few days, or even weeks if necessary, so that you can confidently work your way up the list until you experience no feelings of guilt or anxiety with any of it. You should now be able to incorporate the highest item on your list right from the start of the fantasy, or hold out on yourself so that you prolong the pleasure as you climb the points on your list step by tantalizing step.

This same skill can also be used in real life to overcome anxiety-inducing sexual games or techniques that you or your partner would like to play, but which make you anxious or guilty. In this way you can rehearse in fantasy almost anything one or the other of you wants to try in reality and can come to terms with it gently, under your own control, before trying it out for real. You may find that rehearsing it in fantasy is as far as you feel safe with. If this is so, share this with your partner and agree to restrict the whole subject to your fantasy life for the time being.

SHARING FANTASIES

A recent study found that men who believe they have similar fantasies to those of their partners have the highest numbers of fantasies; and that men who ignore the fantasies of their partners have the lowest fantasy scores. It could be that the men in this study were 'given permission' by their partners' fantasy life to give full rein to their own. Or it could be that knowing that their partners fantasized about much the same things reduced their guilt level. Whatever the explanation, it is a common finding among sexual and marital therapists that couples who are at ease with one another's fantasies have very rich sexual lives and a degree of openness that other couples envy.

Anyone who has come this far in the book will be aware that fantasies reveal a lot about the psyche. For this reason, the sharing of fantasies is rather difficult, calls for a considerable degree of trust, and once done cannot be undone. People find it difficult to open up about their sexual fantasies, even in my therapy sessions, and I have a 'clean' relationship with them, uncluttered by marriage, family, ongoing relationship, and so on. For many people their sexual fantasies are just about the most secret area of their lives and they are loath to share them. Others are even more unwilling to share the fact that they don't have them, for fear of appearing sexually naïve or inept.

In the therapy room things are highly controlled and professional enquiry leads, hopefully, to advantages for the patient. Once an individual starts on the road to fantasy exploration as part of therapy, I find that things improve very quickly, as this very personal area of my client's life is exposed to the light. The considerable harvest of insight that then occurs can take the whole therapy onward in a way that few other single manoeuvres do.

I believe that any caring, loving couple who truly trust one another can do much the same for each other. Many of my patients are terrified of saying anything about their fantasies for fear of being thought perverted or odd in some way. Their own view of themselves often frightens them more than any supposed view their partners might have of them. And this is something that any couple can help one another with. Voicing your fantasies can help make them seem less intimidating, odd, perverted, strange, unacceptable or whatever you might fear they are. They are also, of course, a powerful way for your partner to obtain a deep knowledge of your unconscious.

But sharing fantasies is no easy matter. There is only one valid reason for sharing and that is to enrich and improve the relationship. Revealing your fantasies on the basis that this is how you are and your partner had better know about it can be very dangerous, manipulative and intimidating. The only way to proceed is with considerable caution. If in doubt, say nothing. The thing to remember is that just because something seems OK and perfectly natural to you doesn't necessarily mean that your partner will find it equally so. By jumping in thoughtlessly you could find that you have put your partner off sharing for weeks or even years.

The other thing I find it helpful to point out to my couples is that once you know something about your partner, you can't unknow it. Sometimes a partner whose ideas and attitudes appear terribly up to the minute can be horrified at fantasy revelations the other thought quite tame. On other occasions a partner will mistake a fantasy for a desire to make something happen. This is why I always tell couples that if they have fantasies about people they know in real life (as opposed to film or pop stars, for example) they should keep them to themselves unless their relationship is very strong. If things are excellent between you, it is possible with advantage to share erotic fantasies about people who you know and, in this way, to defuse anything happening in reality. However, most people fear that fantasy could lead to reality, given even a little encouragement. This can be dangerous ground.

I explained in Part One that not all fantasies are unfulfilled wishes. They may be at the very deepest levels of the psyche, but there's usually quite a gulf from there to real life for most people. Many also fantasize about things that are larger than life. A woman who, for example, would like to be taken much more forcibly during sex than her man currently does might fantasize about being 'raped', but wouldn't wish to be raped by him, or, indeed, by anybody in real life. It is these mixed and confusing messages that can make sharing fantasies so difficult.

Once fantasies are shared, the subject of acting them out is never very far behind. One major problem with acting out fantasies is that by doing so, their value can be lost. This is not always so, but many people say it is. In fantasy life everything is perfect and is all geared up to creating the best possible sexual arousal. Once two people start to share a fantasy it loses, or can lose, some of its piquancy; some people say that a fantasy shared, let alone acted out, is never quite the same again. I find that this can be overcome by sharing the fantasy, but not in its entirety or not in its minute detail. Each reader will find an individual answer to this one, according to how much the telling affects the personal value of the fantasy.

By sharing or acting out, couples can also enhance their fantasies. I teach my clients to learn sexy whispering games. In these, the couple takes a favourite fantasy of one partner and the two weave it intricately into their love-making by whispering a story about it as they make love. The details can be varied slightly every time to keep it fresh, but the underlying theme is always one that came originally from the partner's fantasy story. Most recipients of this sort of whispering game are thrilled that their partner not only accepts their fantasy but has taken the trouble to enrich and enhance it while they make love. Most such stories improve in the telling ... especially by the right person, and things get even better as the partner extends the original thread to weave a more exciting tapestry than the originator of the fantasy thought possible.

This brings me to the interesting finding that many couples who are sexually attuned to one another and have well suited personalities have much the same, or complementary, fantasies. Many times I talk with each partner separately, only to find that, unbeknown to either, they have exactly the same, or complementary, fantasies. In my experience this occurs most commonly in couples composed of a man who has rather 'sadistic' fantasies and a woman who has somewhat 'masochistic' ones. They got together originally because they were well matched in their personalities and are often delighted to find that their fantasies match up too. This leads to great richness in their fantasy life, whether or not they ever act anything out in reality.

But all this sharing shouldn't lead to anyone having to act out their fantasies if they don't feel good about doing so. I touched on page 133 on the situation in which some men, and not a few women, say, 'If you really loved me you'd do (whatever it is)'. This puts considerable pressure on the receiver either to make things happen or to appear unloving. Some people even put their whole relationship on the line by expecting their partner to do something about their fantasy, once declared. Sometimes such people are trying to test the relationship on the basis that someone who really loved them would do anything they wanted. But this isn't a viable test of a relationship, because the other may not see the matter under discussion as being any sort of realistic test at all. As one woman put it to me, 'Not wanting to dress up as a whore and have sex doesn't for one moment mean that I don't love him. It's ridiculous'.

So with all of these cautions in front of you, how can you start to share your fantasies with your partner? Straight questioning can work if you know one another well and are aroused at the time. Choose your moment, preferably when you are feeling sexy and starting to make love. Then, gently ask, or reveal something about yourself. Watch for your partner's reaction and back off if there's any sign of a problem. If you want to go by a more roundabout route, how about looking out for what your partner reads, or finds interesting on TV, or in films or videos. Having obtained some ideas, weave them into a fantasy story as you make love, and see how it goes down.

Reading the sexy letters in men's magazines together can be a good source of fantasy talk. Even quite a shy partner will probably open up a little with help. Writing the script outline for an X-rated video, as I suggested on page 151, can work wonders. Here, though, each partner creates a story and then hands it over to the other to read in private. This is a good way to learn about one another's fantasies.

As you will have seen from Part Two, there is much to be learned from the sharing of fantasies. How you interpret them will, of course, depend on your whole relationship and how well you know your partner. It would be foolish to jump to conclusions about the personality of a relatively new partner from the sharing of one fantasy on an early date. It could seriously mislead you about your partner's personality and annoy him or her. However, over some months you should, with intelligence and humility, be able to piece together a more complete picture of your partner's sexuality from his or her fantasy life.

As your insight deepens you can use your new-found knowledge to enhance your physical sex life. Talking your partner through a fantasy might help reduce anxiety, guilt, or whatever negative emotion accompanies it; you can also enhance its value by enriching it, as I have explained. You could also rehearse in fantasy things you intend to do together one day in reality; or create fantasy stories that enable you to deal with one another's sexual needs, which one or other of you will never want to act out. This could help both of you come to terms with some of the practical matters surrounding the new activity. Some fantasies are never going to be acted out, perhaps because they are so fantastic

She has shared her fantasy with her lover and now they relax together after the sex that followed. The sharing has enhanced their intimacy.

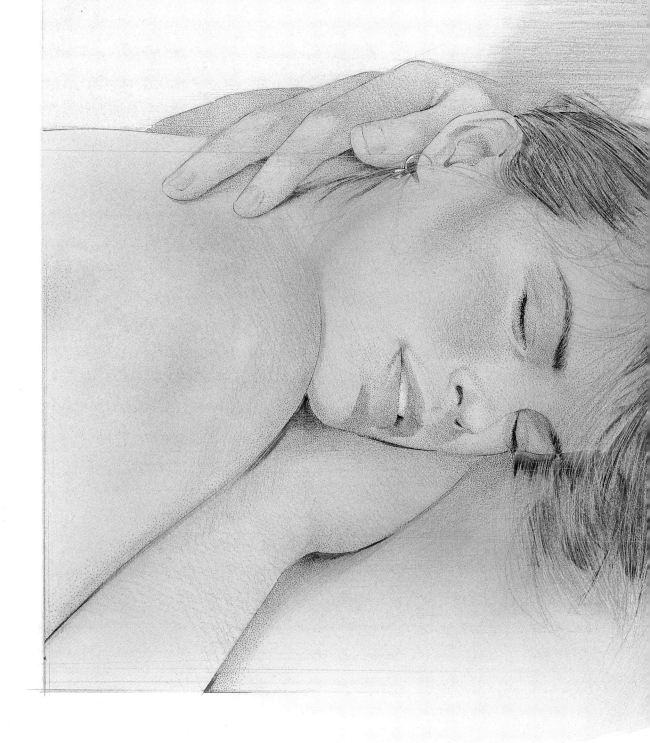

they could never be. In this sort of case the woman could, for example, talk her man through making love to a famous film star while really making love with her. For the keen couple this game can be enhanced by dressing the parts.

I sometimes find that individuals become upset because they have fantasies that distress them. By sharing these, it is possible to get one partner to modify the unacceptable fantasy by changing it slowly over some weeks and whispering, during sex, a different and more acceptable version to the other. A woman client of mine was troubled by having sexual thoughts of her father having sex with her. She had been sexually abused as a little girl and could become highly aroused only if she thought of her father having sex with her.

Her husband was patient and long-suffering over all of this and I suggested that he try to modify her arousal by inserting increasing amounts of more acceptable fantasy material into his sexy stories to her as she neared orgasm. After some months she was able to have a whole fantasy without any of the sex with her father rearing its head. Of course, other work was necessary to help her deal with her sexual abuse, but this bedroom game assisted her as she progressed toward extinguishing the fantasies which, because they were unacceptable to her, got in the way of her pleasure with her husband.

Using a partner's fantasies can be beneficial, in that it can help revive the flagging penis and enrich what would have otherwise been a poor orgasm.

Most couples who know about one another's fantasies can act as sex therapists to one another, as they gain experience of one another's moods and sexual desires.

But for all these positive advantages there are people who see any shared fantasy as something akin to adultery. Some people tell me that while they are aware that both they and their partner fantasize, they would rather not know anything much about it on the grounds that it constitutes some sort of adultery, and might even appear to condone real adultery if they were to be too permissive. Adultery in the mind is clearly a tricky subject for some. In the most profound psychic sense, thinking about having sex with someone is much the same as doing it. In fact, many people are more aroused at the thought of sex with someone else than by the fact of sex with their partner, or, indeed, with their fantasy partner. Many women, especially, tell of their frequent use of fantasy during sexual intercourse for this reason.

However, it is my belief that within a loving, caring relationship such psychic adultery is usually acceptable to the parties involved, provided that it enriches the relationship. After all, there is in fact no danger from any other party in a fantasy affair. Nobody ever caught a sexually transmitted disease from such affairs, nor got pregnant as a result of one.

Other members of the opposite sex don't go away because a couple make a promise of sexual fidelity. I find that fantasy is a highly acceptable way of dealing with such realities in a one-to-one relationship. Couples who pretend that there are no sexual threats to their love bond are starry-eyed optimists who are, in my clinical experience, the ones most likely to cause hurt or be hurt as real life unfolds before them. The successful couple openly acknowledges the attraction of others and accommodates such erotic realities into their sexual and romantic lives.

For such a couple, infidelity in fantasy is a somewhat academic notion, because it serves the relationship's best interests instead of harming it. And in an age when 'till death us do part' is 52 years on average, most people need all the help they can give one another to stay faithful in fact, if not in fantasy. Real life infidelity by definition involves deceit and betrayal. Fantasy affairs that are shared involve neither.

The sharing of fantasies, then, can be one of the most intimate and loving things lovers can do. Most people will choose to do this only once or twice in a lifetime with someone very special. And so it should be. Fantasies come from the very heart of the personality – the depths of the unconscious. And it is these depths that we get together to share in a long-term, love-bonded life together.

Sharing fantasies builds trust between a couple. For some people it beats having sex hands down for intimacy and depth of commmunication. This soul-to-soul sharing brings a couple together in a way that nothing else can. In fact, I find myself professionally wary of the couple who will not do so. They often need to work on their ability to trust, to be intimate and to share in other areas of their life if they are to be happy and successful together.

Clearly, this level of communication and sharing isn't for everybody, but I hope that as a result of reading this book a few more will find true intimacy, love and understanding in their relationship.

INDEX

The page numbers in the index are coded as follows: a number in bold type (**16**) refers to a page on which a fantasy is recounted. A number in italic type (*16*) refers you to a captioned illustration. A number in roman type (16) refers you to a discussion or description in the main text.

WOULD YOU LIKE TO HELP?

Over the many years that I have been interested in erotic fantasies I have had two main sources of information. The first is my patients, who come to see me because of sexual, relationship or marital problems. The second is the learned literature in medical and psychological journals.

Much of the latter originates from the USA. This means that I, and other professionals like me, have very limited direct evidence of what different people in countries all over the world fantasize about.

I would be pleased to hear from any reader about his or her fantasies so that I can gather them together and create a truly international collection. This will be of enormous value in helping to understand how different peoples in different cultures use sexual fantasy. Please send your fantasy to me at the address below.

Dr Andrew Stanway
Eddison Sadd Editions
St Chad's Court
146B King's Cross Road
London WC1X 9DH